A Doc Who Jots*

The more you know about your patient's Story......

William T. Sheahan, MD

* Briefly records stories

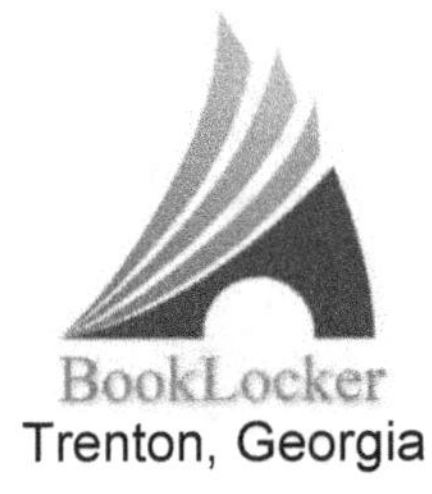

BookLocker
Trenton, Georgia

For Ellie and Tom

Their mom died unexpectedly in 2015. Both were home on a summer break from college at the time. They continue to honor her memory with their character, resilience, and by living life to the fullest.

Giving Thanks

I'm thankful for Veterans.

My dad was an Army Veteran.

My wife is an Air Force Veteran.

Multiple other family members, friends, and acquaintances have served.

Any proceeds generated from this book will be donated to the Fisher House Foundation.

Started in 1990, this foundation builds comfort homes, at major military and Veteran (VA) medical centers, where military and veteran families can stay free of charge, while their loved one is in the hospital receiving treatment.

The Fisher House Foundation has received an A+ rating from Charity Watch, a national charity watchdog service.

Contents

Introduction

Getting to know the whole patient is a core principle of both family medicine and geriatrics—it's especially emphasized during the physician-in-training years.

After medical school I completed a three-year family medicine residency and then a two-year geriatric fellowship.

Once practicing full time, however, my primary focus was to navigate as quickly as possible through encounters, trying to be as productive as the other well-established practitioners in the group.

But envisioning this as my status-quo for years to come, didn't necessarily inspire me to covet a long career in primary care.

I occasionally daydreamed about walking away from medicine for an alternative career even though I had only been out of medical school for about ten years.

However, an article in 1996 by George S. Poehlman MD in *The Journal of Family Practice*, *Dr. Poehlman's pearls*, reminded me of a core principle I had ignored:

"Always ask your patients about something that is totally nonmedical before closing out the patient encounter. You will ensure that your life's work is made up of more than simply treating disease. You will become an amateur anthropologist on whom people's stories are bestowed. This is what makes men and women of medicine wise."

It didn't add a significant amount of time to an encounter, and I started to briefly jot down parts of encounters that seemed unique, uplifting, or funny.

Occasionally, after some reflection, I would also tease out something positive from what may have otherwise been a less-than-optimal encounter.

Behavioralist's refer to this as cognitive reframing.

I had a renewed appreciation for my career, and I transitioned home in a much better frame of mind.

The first three books compiled were entitled "*Patients Say the Darndest Things.*"

(BookLocker.com: book #1: 2003, book #2: 2006, book #3: 2009.)

This collection has a different title.

Surveys have consistently documented that up to fifty percent or more of medical students, residents, nurses, and doctors experience burn out.

It's usually been taught that it's best to avoid getting too close to patients emotionally to reduce the risk for burn out.

It's logical to think this way for self-preservation and to ensure professional boundaries are maintained.

However, in their book, *Compassionomics*, Drs. Trzeciak and Mazzarelli present evidence-based information that contrasts with this previously accepted dogma:

"*Compassion is not only a powerful therapy for the person receiving compassion, but it is a powerful therapy for the person giving compassion too. That's what the latest science shows. And that's why compassion can be such a powerful treatment for burnout among health care providers.*"

"Of course, it is intuitive to some extent that there could be risk of burnout with repeated or excessive exposure to human suffering. However, the preponderance of data in the scientific literature supports a different view: It shows that human connection can transform the experience for the giver of compassion, trigger positive emotion, and build resilience."

Health is not necessarily the absence of disease--It's a state of mind that allows a person to remain resilient--to enjoy and appreciate life to the greatest extent possible--despite his or her underlying medical diagnoses or conditions.

It's therefore feasible that resilience can be enhanced in both the provider and the patient through increased human connectiveness.

Pastor Rick Warren has noted that a key to improving most relationships is to *"Don't try to be interesting; be interested."*

Parker Palmer has said, *"The more you know about another person's story, the less possible it is to see that person as your enemy."*

I've amended his quote to *"The more you know about your patient's story, the less possible it is to see that person as just your patient."*

Sadly, suicide rates for health care workers are significantly higher than the general population, while many health indices are lower.

Fortunately, most healthcare organizations now have dedicated teams to promote wellness. Some even have "chief wellness officers," many of whom are physicians.

There are also independent practices around the country that offer retreats, conferences, consultations, and counseling for health care professionals in need.

It's been shown that there's a direct correlation between wellness and job satisfaction, work attendance, retention, revenues, quality of care and patient satisfaction scores.

Some thoughts on difficult patient encounters.

Clinicians rate a high percentage of encounters with patients as difficult.

It's often not difficult in the sense of having complex medical issues; it's just being difficult, for a multitude of reasons, which includes aberrant behavior.

Recent surveys have concluded that aberrant behavior has, unfortunately, increased during the pandemic.

Most practitioners note a greater degree of disillusionment with their medical career after experiencing numerous such encounters.

An encounter that invokes less than altruistic thoughts is usually consistent with my definition of a difficult encounter.

The late Dr. B. Lewis Barnett, Jr., was a mentor, a friend, and a family medicine icon. In his book, *"Between the Lines (Reflections of a Family Physician),"* Dr. B. noted, *"There are patients who try our souls and who seem to be the devil's very advocate,"* but then also reminds us that we must *"look through the dismal side of them to see their real beauty and worth."*

Clinicians are more likely to consider encounters as difficult when they are defensive, angry, arrogant, authoritative, sleep deprived, or burnt-out.

My attitude and biases can also play a significant role in less-than-optimal encounters.

Therefore, it's appropriate to self-reflect on my role in either contributing to or exacerbating difficult encounters.

Behavioral experts offer advice through books, articles, conferences, and role play but experience, including many less-than-optimal encounters, has enlightened me as to which strategies seem to work most consistently.

Staying calm, remaining as respectful as possible, and showing empathy, has been my most successful formula.

And, getting difficult patients to also engage about something that is totally nonmedical, if such efforts are possible and not rebuked, may help to foster a more favorable relationship over time.

Negative thoughts on my part may then be considerably attenuated.

Compliance also typically improves—so many chronic conditions become more manageable--often without any other significant interventions.

As a result, many days of patient care are much better than they would have been otherwise.

Finally, remember to acknowledge that there's nothing quite like being a patient.

You're fortunate if you haven't been a patient to any significant extent.

I have been several times.

This role reversal is humbling but has always increased my empathy and understanding for the plight of my patients.

My Doc Jots

The COVID-19 pandemic has profoundly impacted us all.

The encounters herein were prior to the pandemic. All but a handful are encounters with patients at the office or at their homes, and many of the stories will have little to do with the reason for the medical appointment.

The patients are primarily middle-aged and elderly.

All the names (or initials) of the patients have been changed.

Some have since died.

Many family medicine docs have cared for all ages of patients throughout their career; some have even continued to do deliveries. I hold most all of them in the highest of regard.

My career path resulted in a narrower patient demographic.

Many encounters do not have as pleasant an outcome as depicted on many of the pages that follow.

However, some will illustrate the ability to tease out a positive feature from what may have otherwise been a less-than-optimal encounter.

Some personal reflections are included at the end, with a couple sections on navigating through grieving and bereavement after experiencing a sudden, unexpected loss.

It's better late than never.

I saw Mr. P., a white man, shortly after his 50th birthday.

He let me know he was planning to finally start taking better care of himself now that he was middle-aged.

He had not been one of my more compliant patients over the years.

I smiled, told him that was great to hear, but then decided to question, "By the way, how many 100-year-old men do you know?"

He looked confused.

Mr. P.: I don't know any.

Me: There are some but the current average life span for an American white male is 76-77 years, so we both may have been middle-aged when we were about 38 years old.

Mr. P.: Well, that's a bummer.

Me: No, I don't look at it that way. It's just a good reminder that life comes at us fast and it's never too late to start taking better care of yourself.

He smiled and sort of agreed with me.

Putting things in perspective.

A 25-year-old man was concerned about "tiny bumps on his penis."

His exam was notable for the complete absence of body and pubic hair.

He did not have alopecia universalis.

He just spent a lot of time in the shower with a razor or at a hair waxing salon.

An exam of his penis revealed Tyson's glands.

Tyson's glands are tiny sebaceous (oil) glands, are considered normal, and are completely harmless.

I spent a fair amount of time trying to reassure him that all was fine.

He questioned how he could go through the rest of his life deformed.

He questioned how he could ever be intimate with someone in the future.

He was not completely satisfied with my explanation, even after showing him pictures from dermatology and patient education sites.

A colleague is a dermatologist in the next building.

He offered to see him and do a quick curbside consultation.

He agreed with my assessment.

He also did not recommend any specific treatment, only reassurance.

Finally, the patient asked the dermatologist, "Isn't there some way to get rid of them permanently."

"Yes," he replied, "amputate your penis."

After a brief pause, we all laughed.

"I guess it's not so bad after all," he said.

I didn't mean for that to happen!

I have been following a 54-year-old man for many years. He has the usual assortment of medical diagnoses. He also smokes 1-2 packs a day.

I had previously tried many different approaches to get him to quit smoking.

No idea why on this day, a routine follow-up appointment, I decided to ask, "Are your wife and other family members prepared to meet your needs after you've had a heart attack or a stroke?"

He smiled, then laughed and said, "Yes they are, good try, Doc."

He was still not ready to quit. We spent time talking about the trip he was about to make up north to see other family members.

Unfortunately, I received a phone call message about a week later. He was still away on vacation.

"Let Doc know he was right. I had a heart attack and a stroke and am still in the hospital. My heart is doing okay, but I don't have a lot of movement on my left side."

I have seen him in the office since. He has quit smoking. He still has considerable left sided weakness. His family is helping to meet his needs.

He thinks I'm smarter than I am just because I predicted his future.

It has not changed my desire to get folks to quit smoking, just the phraseology I use with other patients.

Stop talking so much!

A 61-year-old man came in for a follow-up appointment.

Me: Good to see you. Anything new?

Patient: We've been doing a lot of traveling lately.

Me: That's excellent, do you go by car, or do you have an RV?

Patient: We have an RV.

Me: That's great.

I then decided to go on a long tangent reminiscing about growing up with my dad selling RVs, taking family trips in RVs, having a job cleaning the RV rental fleet, and how the gas crisis in the mid-1970s crushed the business for many years. I enjoyed reminiscing. The patient did not seem to mind.

Finally, I stopped to catch my breath.

Me: So how did everything go locating RV parks while you were traveling?

Patient: What do you mean?

Me: Didn't you need to plan to make sure there would be an RV park wherever you stopped for the day?

Patient: We would have if we took the RV. These last trips we always went in our car. We stayed in hotels.

Me: Oh...that's cool.

I've got to stop talking so much!

Mr. G's longevity recipe.

I always enjoy seeing Mr. G.; I've known him for close to 13 years.

He has what others might term a cantankerous personality.

He's an 88-year-old who lives in the country, is a nudist, smokes, chews tobacco, and drinks excessively.

He has a history of hypertension, coronary heart disease, congestive heart failure, peripheral vascular disease, and emphysema.

He remains completely independent. He walks without a cane or walker. He's cognitively intact. He's continent.

He's compliant with his medications.

He's been married for 54 years, but he and his wife have lived in separate homes, on the same piece of property, for the last 20 years or so.

Me: Are you still using your special recipe every morning?

Patient: You bet, as regular as a goose going barefooted.

Me: Can you review it for me again?

Patient: Yep, I drink a V-8, followed by 2 beers, then 3 cups of coffee, one more beer, eat a raw onion and then have 2-3 cigars.

Over the course of a typical day, he smokes 5-7 cigars, drinks 6-9 beers and chews tobacco. His favorite food, beside onions, are his "beans and weenies."

Patient: Go ahead Doc, get it over with...

Me: You shouldn't be smoking cigars, chewing tobacco, or drinking so much.

He laughs...and I can't keep from smiling.

His clinical exam remains incredibly stable. At the end of most visits, he always makes sure to remind me of one thing.

Patient: Don't see many folks my age doing as well as I am, do you?

Me: Nope, I don't, see you in about 6 months.

The Dancing Man.

Health is not the absence of disease. It's the state of mind that lets one live a full, rewarding, and productive life regardless of their physical condition. Mr. C. was a perfect example.

He had more than his fair share of medical conditions over the years: hypertension, COPD, prostate cancer, colon cancer, recurrent deep venous thromboses, severe peripheral vascular disease and end stage degenerative joint disease.

He lived with his daughter and son-in-law. He loved to dance.

Every Friday and Saturday he had the same routine:

He would dress up and then take a cab to arrive at his dancing establishment by 8 PM. He would take the cab so as not to burden his family, even though they always offered to drive him. He would dance until around 1 AM with the support of his partners, and his walker. From there he would go for coffee at Denny's and then take the cab home at 3-4 AM.

His daughter had questions:

Was it okay for him to continue to do this?

Was she doing the right thing letting her father do this?

He really seems to want to do this, doesn't he?

My response: Yes, yes, and yes.

He was a great example of health, despite his physical condition.

I smile every time I think about him.

The PG-rated version of a common primary care topic.

I spend a fair amount of time reviewing issues concerning erectile dysfunction (ED) with men. It's still interesting that, despite all the information available, many are still so uninformed on many of the issues involved.

What follows are some things I try and review with patients.

1. If you want to perform like Tarzan, you must feel like the king of the jungle. Therefore, if you are not confident in your ability to perform, for whatever reason, there will often be dysfunction.

2. If everything works while you are alone, your plumbing and hydraulics are intact.

3. If you are not physically and/or emotionally attracted to your partner, your chance of success is less.

4. The heavily advertised, and commonly prescribed, oral medications do not work by themselves. In other words, you can't take one and then stare down and wait for things to rise on their own.

5. If you are in a relationship that does not have respectful communication at its core your chance of ED is greater.

6. If you are in a relationship in which you are not yet comfortable to talk about ED with each other, you should wait until you are prior to trying to be intimate. See #7.

7. If you are not able to tell your partner that you are using medical treatments to assist with ED, it's probably not a strong enough relationship yet.

8. Four of the best things to do, if applicable (even better if you do it together): stop smoking, limit alcohol, lose weight and exercise. See #9.

9. Smoking, excessive alcohol use, being overweight and lack of exercise are probably more the cause of ED than the low dose of blood pressure or anti-depressant medication you are taking.

10. Something as simple as a retention ring, available on the internet without a prescription, might be enough to allow you to perform for all to be happy. A vacuum pump is also a good nonpharmacologic choice.

11. A low Testosterone level may play a role in a few, especially if you lack desire.

12. Remember that satisfaction, as a couple, does not always need to include "the act."

13. Success can almost always be achieved; it just depends on how much intervention one is willing to accept. Most clinics that guarantee success do so with the aid of a syringe and needle.

I usually let patients know that I would prefer to do numbers 1-12 before considering number 13. Most, who are willing to take part in the discussion, agree.

A preventative health reminder in a nice color.

A 58-year-old man came in for a new patient appointment. He was wearing a bright blue rubber bracelet on his wrist that had the statement "Colon Cancer Screening Saves Lives."

I read it aloud while I was checking his pulse.

Me: Colon cancer screening saves lives.

Patient: I'm sorry, what?

Me: Colon cancer screening saves lives.

Patient: Oh, colon cancer screening saves lives?

Me: Yes, just like your bracelet says.

Patient: Oh (now looking down at his wrist), that's cool. I've never really paid any attention to what was written on it. I've just always liked the color. Someone gave it to me about a year ago.

We then talked about a screening colonoscopy since he never had one before.

He agreed to be referred for one.

Wow…that bracelet worked great!

From your nose?

A staff member called to let me know she had been vomicking all night and would not be into work.

I've heard this from patients over the years, just never from a health care professional.

I've always just assumed vomicking was being substituted for the correct word, vomiting.

However, it's listed in the urban dictionary.

"The act of spewing forth your stomach contents from your nose."

Yikes…is all I can say for those who are truly vomicking and not just vomiting!

Huff the magic dragon.

The staff at the ALF suspected Mr. L. was huffing by using a computer dusting product.

When called with their concern, I was luckily able to quickly look up what huffing meant!

He denied it on multiple occasions, but the staff eventually caught him asleep with the straw of the duster literally still up his nose.

The chemical in the duster, difluoroethane, has significant CNS effects and is highly addictive.

This was a new one for me.

Hopefully we can get him some help.

Drive-by inspiration

On the way to a home visit, I passed a small rural church that had the following message on their sign:

"Aspire to Inspire before you Expire."

I'm trying…

Senior texting acronyms

My brother shared some senior texting acronyms with me. Here are a few of my favorites:

ATDs-at the doctor's
BTW-bring the wheelchair
BYOT-bring your own teeth
GGPBL-gotta go, pacemaker battery low

HGBM-had good bowel movement
OMINJG-oh my, it's not just gas
TOT-texting on toilet
WFA-wet furniture again
WTP-where're the prunes

Men of few words.

Some doctors are men of few words.

I had carpal tunnel surgery a few years ago.

On my initial follow-up I was asked how everything was going.

Me: Okay, but my fingers are still numb.

Orthopedic surgeon: The incision looks fine.

Me: But my fingers are still numb.

Orthopedic surgeon: Thanks for coming in (as he walked out the door).

I saw the same surgeon a year later for a different concern.

Me: …but my hand is finally doing well. It took about 6 months for the numbness to go away.

Orthopedic surgeon: Just like I told you. Thanks for coming in (as he walked out the door).

Psychic powers.

Warning: The following brief patient encounter confirms I'm easily amused, often finding humor in things that most "normal" folks would not.

A 78-year-old man came in for an appointment after undergoing several tests by his cardiologist.

Me: How did everything turn out?

(I hadn't yet received any information concerning the results.)

Patient: I have a premonition that everything is fine.

(Quick review-premonition: An intuition of a future occurrence; a feeling; a hunch; a warning in advance; a forewarning; an early warning of a future event; a feeling of anticipation of or anxiety over a future event.)

Me: Why's that?

Patient: Well, the cardiologist was sitting in the room while all the tests were being done (an EKG, an echocardiogram, and a nuclear stress test). He made the comment, a few times, that everything looked excellent and that my heart was in great shape for a 78-year-old man.

Me: That sounds like a pretty good premonition.

Later that morning his psychic powers were confirmed. The faxed results received confirmed all the tests were normal.

I still think it's funny!

A life outside of the medical office.

I've known Mr. F. for a long time.

He has chronic pain from degenerative joint disease, as well as multiple other medical and psychiatric diagnoses.

Every time I see him, he appears miserable.

I always try, as I do with all folks with chronic pain, to have as much empathy as possible.

Recently, my wife, son, daughter, and I went to see a movie.

It was a comedy. We got to our seats during the coming attractions, so the theater was already dark.

After my eyes adjusted, I noticed that Mr. F. was sitting in the row directly in front of ours. I didn't say anything to him, and it didn't appear that he noticed me (I often wear a baseball cap when not at work).

During the movie he was, at times, laughing loudly at the parts in which everyone else in the theater was laughing.

I found myself watching him more than the movie.

It was wonderful to see this person, who usually appears almost lifeless in my office, smiling and, at times, laughing hysterically. I had never seen him so animated.

It was great to see!

It was uplifting.

He seemed to be enjoying himself, and for at least this brief two-hour span, life itself.

He left as soon as the movie ended. We waited until most of the credits were finished.

I've seen him since.

I haven't let him know I saw him outside of the office. It doesn't change the fact that he has chronic pain. It just sort of gives me feedback that he's doing a little better emotionally, and possibly physically, than I had thought.

I really wanted to tap him on the shoulder during the movie and say, "it's good to see you and thanks for making me feel better about how you are doing!"

Thanks for the feedback.

A patient filled out a complaint form asking to leave my practice and gave it to my office administrator.

I was asked to "sign-off" on the complaint (as is always our practice).

It said that he wanted to transfer to another doctor, since I always spent time telling him about my problems.

I had no comment since I wasn't sure what he was talking about.

It just so happened that, soon after requesting to transfer, he came in for an acute medical concern and my partner (whom he had transferred to) was on vacation.

It was, admittedly, a little awkward seeing him but I remained professional.

At the end of the visit he said, "Thanks for seeing me, I hope you weren't offended that I asked to transfer to your partner."

I saw my opening. "Not at all, I was just a little confused by the comment that I was always telling you about my problems. I didn't know what you meant."

"The last time I came to see you and was concerned about a mole, you told me it was nothing to worry about and then pulled up your pant leg to show me you had the same type of mole (a seborrheic keratosis). The visit before that I was concerned about a bump under my skin, and you pulled up your shirt sleeve to show me you had the same thing on your arm (a lipoma)."

"Oh, okay, thanks for the feedback."

I learn something new every day.

I'll probably not change the way I interact with folks.

I'll just always wonder if someone else is thinking the same thing, whenever I show them some of my own physical exam findings, while trying to reassure them.

Trying to prevent fires (in the office).

All it takes for a health care provider to have increased empathy for patients is to have a health-related concern of his/her own, or within his/her family. That way providers can experience the many communication deficiencies in our health care system.

Many times, a statement made during a patient encounter can help to establish or re-establish a relationship that might have been lost.

Things obviously don't always go smoothly in the office. Occasionally, I resort to a couple of old standbys to help defuse a tension filled room. Both have withstood the test of time, for the most part.

* When seeing a new patient who appears (by his body language/facial expression) to be upset, angry, disillusioned, etc., by the medical system: "You look upset. I'm sorry. I don't think we've ever met before. It's good to meet you. I'll certainly try to do everything I can to help assist with your medical needs and to be your advocate."

* When an encounter has, for whatever reason, deteriorated to almost a point of no return: "Would it be alright if we started over. I'm sorry that things got off to a bad start. I apologize. Let's start over, okay?"

The most expensive care anywhere.

A 32-year-old man had been to the emergency room (ER) in the community for lower abdominal discomfort.

He brought a copy of his records with him.

His abdominal exam was noted as being benign. No other significant physical exam was done.

Labs (blood and urine), as well as an abdominal and pelvic CT scan were normal.

No diagnosis or treatment was given.

He was told to see his primary care provider the next day.

As part of his exam the next day, palpation of the epididymis of one testicle caused significant pain in his testicle and lower abdomen.

He had epididymitis. He was involved in a long-term monogamous relationship.

He was told to use underwear with more support and given a prescription for a $3 generic antibiotic.

A week later, on re-check, he was fine (cured!).

He had already received one bill from the ER for approximately $2200.00.

Additional bills from the emergency room visit would surely be arriving soon.

You gotta laugh!

A 63-year-old man has advanced Parkinson's-Plus Syndrome. He has significant rigidity, immobility, falls often and has not responded favorably to most medication trials.

His daughter (his caregiver) came with him to the appointment.

It was a sad encounter as they were recalling the most recent visit to a neurologist who was an expert in neurodegenerative diseases. I hadn't received the consult note back yet.

The patient was teary eyed when he let me know the neurologist said there was "nutin more he could do."

After a brief pause, I responded, "He really said that?"

"Yes."

"He said nutin...n-u-t-i-n?"

Thankfully, all thought it was funny and laughed.

Laughter's still the best medicine!

Definition #1, I think.

While taking a social history on an elderly male:

Patient: ...and my son Boo-Boo lives just around the corner and comes to see how we are doing at least every other day.

Me: Your son is named Boo-Boo?

(Quick definition: #1. A stupid or embarrassing mistake; a blunder or #2. A slight physical injury, such as a scratch)

Patient: My wife and I planned to have two children, but we had three and he's the youngest, so it's always been his nickname.

Me: Wow, that's a little harsh, but funny! How old is he now?

Patient: He just turned 65.

A great start to a day in the office.

An 82-year-old man was born on September 5th.

He just so happened to have the first appointment of the day with me on a September 5th.

I noticed his date of birth just prior to going into the exam room to see him.

I grabbed a small candy bar from our office secret stash and gave it to him when I entered the exam room.

Me: Happy birthday! I'm sorry I couldn't put a candle in the candy bar.

Patient: Thanks. You know some years my birthday falls on Labor Day...of course it was a Labor Day, regardless, for my mother on the year I was born!

He then laughed almost uncontrollably for a bit, and I smiled with him.

It was a great way to start the day.

Later, I couldn't help but think how great it was for him to have this life-long joke that still gave him a bout of laughter every time he got the opportunity to tell it to someone new.

An office yogi-ism (for all Yogi Berra fans).

A 79-year-old man with multiple medical diagnoses:

Patient: Don't get me wrong Doc. I'm grateful to be alive. A lot of my friends, who I hang out with all the time and are my same age, aren't alive anymore.

Me: (After my "what did he just say" pause) You bet, I'm glad you're thankful for good health.

My bad.

I was seeing a 47-year-old patient.

Me: Still smoking two packs a day?

Patient: No (said with an annoyed, somewhat angry tone)!

Me: How much are you smoking now?

Patient: I almost always come in under two packs a day.

Me: So, a pack and a half a day?

Patient: Yeah, on most days.

Me: I'm sorry I assumed you were smoking forty cigarettes a day. It's great to know you're only smoking about thirty a day.

Surprisingly, I then caught the slightest hint of a smile on his face.

Feeling out of balance?

A few years ago, folks with all kinds of musculoskeletal complaints would come in for an appointment due to the same, while wearing magnetic bracelets. Often, if I was feeling particularly devious, I would ask, "Aren't those bracelets supposed to correct your musculoskeletal issues?"

The newest craze are the balance bracelets (a rubber bracelet with a little piece of, what looks like, tinfoil). I'm at a medical conference this weekend and I've even spotted a few health care providers wearing them.

Here's the "scientific" information I could find: "The bracelets contain two hologram's which are embedded with frequencies that react with your body's electromagnetic field. When the power hologram contacts your body's energy field it begins to resonate in accordance with everyone's energy system, creating a harmonic loop that optimizes your energy field. It maintains energy flow while it clears the pathways so electrochemical exchange functions like the well-tuned generator it was designed to be."

Oh, and don't forget the usual disclaimer: "The above statements have not been evaluated by the FDA. This product is not intended to diagnose, treat, cure, or prevent any disease process."

Wow. Can't think of anything else to say.

It just brings up one question, however: why do so many patients have a hard time understanding and accepting why disease entities such as uncontrolled diabetes, hypertension, hypothyroidism, sleep apnea, etc. can affect multiple body systems when they seem so capable of accepting the "science" behind their $29.95 balance bracelets?

Pondering elective orthopedic surgery?

A quick recommendation:

If you are thinking about undergoing an elective orthopedic surgery (knee, hip, back, etc.), do not talk with anyone who is sitting in a doctor's waiting room.

Often, if you do, you may find that it's someone who had the same procedure you are considering having done and who, unfortunately, did not do well.

It's much better to talk with folks you meet shopping, socializing, fishing, golfing, traveling, etc. They are usually in the larger subset of patients that underwent the procedure and had a successful outcome.

Talking with them will allow you to be in a much better frame of mind while weighing the pros and cons of having an elective orthopedic procedure performed.

It's mine!

A 51-year-old man was being seen for the first time for a complete physical exam.

While doing the exam I noticed he had his first name tattooed, length wise, on the shaft of his penis.

He didn't mention anything. I made a comment after pondering what to say when wrapping up our visit.

Me: If your penis ever shows up in a lost and found it will be easy to claim.

He smiled.

Patient: I was just really drunk one night. It's a good thing I didn't have a long name.

We both laughed.

Hallelujah dances.

All practitioners have some difficult patients.

My definition of a difficult patient is simple: it's someone who, for whatever reason, invokes a feeling of dread or doom in you and/or your staff.

It usually has nothing to do with a patients age or their underlying medical diagnoses or co-morbidities. Some are part of your life only briefly; others you get to know for many, many years.

I used to enjoy watching the television show *"Becker."*

The actor, Ted Danson, played the part of an internist (Dr. Becker) working in a New York City medical office.

In one of the episodes, one of his difficult patients announced she was moving south to live with a son.

Dr. Becker then went on to say how much he had enjoyed taking care of her over the years and how much he would miss being her doctor.

He then let the patient know he would be right back and excused himself for a minute. He closed the exam room door.

Once in the hallway and alone, he broke into a huge grin and started to do a "hallelujah" dance.

After this moment of joy, he went back into the exam room and finished his solemn good-byes.

Many primary care providers can understand the joy he temporarily expressed. Just always remember to dance in private.

Get back on your toes, now!

I'm asked to fill out disability forms for patients frequently, but some assessment forms, in my opinion, ask ridiculous questions such as:

During an 8-hour workday, what percentage of time can the individual walk on heels, walk on toes, squat, or crawl?

During an 8-hour workday, what percentage of time can the individual lift 0-4lbs, 5-9lbs, 10-14lbs, 15-19lbs, etc.?

I guess I have an easy job when it comes to physicality.

None of my patients, however, has ever admitted to having to spend part of his/her workday heel or toe walking while carrying weights.

I guess someone must.

The same questions keep appearing.

I would love to be a fly on the wall at their workplace.

Can't help but wonder what kind of job they must have?

Moving to Florida.

I've practiced in central Florida since 1993.

I can't begin to count the number of times I've heard "My doctor up north told me I needed to move to Florida (pronounced Flor-ee-da by many north easterners) to improve my health."

I love Florida and I'm not a fan of the cold and snow, but for some elderly folks I can't help but think:

-Your doctor felt this heat and humidity would be good for your health?

-Your doctor felt that our air quality (high pollen counts, wildfires, etc.) would be good for your health?

-Your doctor felt that moving away from all your extended family members would be beneficial?

Occasionally I think...

What would I use as a reason to "move back up north to improve your health?"

-You could use the warm clothes you still own.

-The cold weather might reduce swelling in certain parts of your body (could be true).

-Being close to other family members, who still live up north, might be beneficial to help in your personal and health care needs (hopefully would be true for many).

and finally...

-You could use your long-term memory to navigate routes and/or remember the names of people and places (from years ago), even when you have short term memory impairments!

Three useful (equestrian) terms.

I spent a good part of this past weekend (and many other parts of weekends) at a horse show.

My 15 y/o daughter has been riding for about 4 years and is an accomplished equestrian.

She rides her horse (Blues) almost every day and they compete in shows at least once a month.

I've picked up a few horse terms over the years that sure encompass a lot:

1. Colic: when something is wrong with the horse's digestive tract-can represent anything from gas to intestinal torsion (life threatening). Luckily, whenever our horse has had colic, a massive passage of gas has always been curative, so far.

2. Lame: means that something is wrong from a musculoskeletal standpoint. It also means that the horse can't

be ridden (a real bummer for my daughter, as well as for those who are writing the checks for her to ride!).

3. Sound: all good. A-okay. Ready for action. Now we're talking!

Three useful terms.

It would make documenting a lot easier if I could use them in office notes for my patients!

Know the number.

Unfortunately, I see patients everyday with horrible teeth.

I keep emergency supplies in my office, so I can brush and floss my own teeth, whenever I finish looking into the mouth of such a patient.

I've received dental consults back over the years with notes concerning work done on tooth #11, #12, #20 and #22, for example.

Finally, after many years, I decided to investigate how teeth are numbered.

The Universal tooth numbering system always starts on the right upper back-the third molar is tooth #1. It continues to the left upper back (third molar #16), then down to the bottom back left (tooth #17) and on around to the right lower back (tooth #32).

Numbers are assigned and remain the same even when a tooth has been pulled.

My knowing this numbering system hasn't done a darn thing in improving the dental hygiene of my patients.

It just makes me feel good about using the dentist's "lingo" when placing a consult or calling a dental colleague over the phone.

I even had one dentist remark that it was rare to have the referring medical provider use the numbering system, but that it was greatly appreciated.

I didn't let him know I was smiling on the other end of the phone.

Look at the watch.

Many elderly folks still wear "old fashioned" watches-not smart watches.

Although there are no studies, I often use the "watch test" as another quick office check for cognitive impairment--even in those who I had not previously suspected of being impaired.

When I check a pulse, as I do on all patients, I always look to see if the watch is right side up and if the time is correct.

The day and date are not as important. My eyes are younger than most of my patients and even I have a hard time reading those on most watches.

If either the orientation or the time is wrong, cognitive impairment is possible.

Putting a watch on every day is part of a long-term routine for most elderly folks.

Having it on correctly and with the correct time involves a higher level of function.

The day after a 91.

Cool story...

Last week I had a first visit with a 60-year-old male. He moved to this area after separating from his wife-this is not the cool part of the story.

He's a golf pro and he's already employed by a country club.

He became a pro at about age 40, after an almost 20-year career as a circulation manager for a major metropolitan newspaper.

I asked if he ever played in a tour event.

Patient: I became a pro because I loved to play, but mainly because I loved to teach. I struggled with wondering if I should try to play on the tour or just continue to be a teaching pro. Finally, I qualified for an event. On the first day, I shot a 51 on the front nine and a 40 on the back nine. A 91 (for all nongolfer's that's 20 over par-a terrible round for a professional)! That night I wanted to quit because I was embarrassed. I then realized it was Gods way of letting me know playing on the tour wasn't for me. I felt this huge sense of relief. The next day I shot a 68 (a very good score; three under par). Obviously, I didn't make the cut for the final two rounds but felt great. I knew what I was supposed to do for the rest of my life: teach golf.

That's the cool part of the story!

An inexpensive nose job.

A 56-year-old man:

Patient: I broke my nose when I was younger and it had a bad curve, but since I've gotten older and started to wear glasses, it straightened out.

Me: You had your nose straightened with surgery?

Patient: No, wearing glasses with the nose pads just seemed to straighten it out.

Me: Okay, that's great (it looked quite straight).

I couldn't think of anything else to say. For the rest of the day, however, I kept taking off my glasses to look at and feel my relatively flimsy nose pads.

I had no idea they were capable of such great feats!

I'm sure the plastic surgeons and ENT doctors will try to keep this from becoming widespread knowledge.

Not so simple.

I was returning a phone call to a 57-year-old patient I had known for years.

Me: How can I help you?

Patient: It's simple. I'm applying for disability. I just need for you to write a brief statement in my record that it's your opinion I contracted hepatitis C from exposure to blood while I was working.

Amid saying, "Oh" and asking "What do you need again?" I quickly found a consult note from an infectious disease (ID) specialist from about 7 years ago. The very first sentence of the note said, "He reports that he did intravenous drugs in the 1970s and feels that's how he was infected."

Me: I'm looking at a note from about seven years ago in your record. Let me read it to you (I then read the ID note word for word to him).

Patient: Oh, I didn't know that was in there. Um, thanks. I'll get back to you later if I have any questions.

Me: You bet.

I then said a silent, "Thank you computerized patient record!"

Medication reconciliation...not.

I see patients all the time who have returned to Florida for the winter months.

It's always great when they bring in copies of their medical records.

Every document now includes medication reconciliation.

What seems to be lacking, however, is a careful review of the medications and the instructions for use.

The computer-generated print outs often look impressive.

Reviews, however, can reveal many errors.

Often, for example, one beta blocker was substituted for another beta blocker, but both still appear on the medication reconciliation sheet.

Obviously, this can lead to adverse medication effects.

Had a nice man recently return from up north, having been hospitalized just prior to returning, for poorly controlled diabetes mellitus.

He was confused as to what dose of insulin he should take.

His medication reconciliation sheet had the following instructions (re-typed exactly as written):

Lantus 100 units/ml subcutaneous solution. Directions for use: 60 units subcutaneous of Lantus at bedtime, decrease to 30 units of Lantus, decrease to 15 units of Lantus, then discontinue Lantus.

The instructions were admittedly hard to understand.

Easy rule: if a health care professional can't understand the instructions, it's appropriate to assume that our patients can't either.

A lot of computer-generated signatures are entered on documents that have not been carefully read. The medication reconciliation page is one that needs to be carefully reviewed before signing.

He's got a valid argument.

An 85-year-old man was new to my practice.

He came to the appointment with his wife.

Wife (during the history): He also needs his memory pills.

Me: What pills does he take?

Wife: Honey, what's the name of your memory pills?

Patient: I don't know. I can't remember. That's a stupid question to ask me, isn't it?

Everyone then laughed.

All in the family.

51-year-old man. He was an attorney.

Me (during the social history): How many children do you have?

Patient: Three. They're all grown and out on their own.

Me: What do they do for a living?

Patient: They all work for me. None of them went to college but they're all real smart. My oldest son helps with bankruptcies. My daughter does investigations for my cases that go into litigation and my youngest son just started with me. He's does background checks and is a whiz with finances. They all do an excellent job. My oldest boy is as skilled in bankruptcy knowledge as any attorney I know. I'm very proud of them.

Me: Let me guess. Does your wife work with you?

Patient: Yeah, she's the office manager.

Me: Do any of them want to become an attorney?

Patient: No. I'm just hoping I can hang in there until one of my grandchildren goes to law school to take over the practice.

Now that's cool!

More than just a brave man.

Reading an obituary on a patient of mine highlighted a missed opportunity.

Mr. D. was an incredibly brave and stoic man.

When I first met him, he had already been diagnosed with three different primary cancers.

He was also being followed at an acclaimed cancer treatment center.

He was on accepted chemotherapy regimens, as well as on some investigational drugs.

In my role as his primary care physician, I was never able to give much insight into his current treatment regimen or guidance regarding some of the various side effects he was experiencing.

I admittedly tried to keep the appointments as brief as possible.

I never really got to know him as more than an unfortunate man with three different primary cancers, who was extremely brave.

I read his obituary yesterday:

"He is survived by his wife of 44 years. He joined the Air Force after high school and was active duty for 4 years. After serving, he went to college, played basketball, broke every offensive record, and was named to the All-America team. He was a successful small business owner and raised two children. His daughter is a teacher, and his son is an attorney."

I wish I would gotten to know him better while he was alive, despite how uncomfortable I was in seeing him.

My lesson re-learned.

Intact social graces.

I got into the habit years ago of noting if a patient with dementia had intact social graces.

By this I mean they can converse and appear pleasant.

I always record this because these are the patients that sometimes need closer follow up to determine if their dementia is advancing.

They tend to be engaging and conversant, even when they can't answer orientation questions, etc.

They answer questions, but the answers frequently don't match the question that was asked.

They also tend to deflect questions by asking their own questions such as "so how are you and your family doing?"

This often causes a provider, such as me, to go on a long tangent to give them a family update.

At times, it's such a pleasant encounter that it's easy to forget they are even demented.

But if I get dementia, I hope my social graces stay intact.

In my experience, it sure makes things a lot easier for the caregiver(s)!

It's true.

Several years ago, I wrote an entry in *Patients Say the Darndest Things,* book #2 entitled, *"Possible antidotes for the primary care blues."*

In one section I asked, "have you been sued lately?"

I noted "a study has shown most physicians report shame, anger, self-doubt and disillusion with their medical career after going through litigation, regardless of the outcome of the suit."

I graduated from medical school in 1985.

At the time I wrote the entry, I had never been sued.

This is no longer the case.

I can now confirm it's a true statement.

Office research.

I have a bad habit of seeking chocolate during a stressful day.

Today someone had placed Peanut M & M's, fun size bags, in our office secret candy stash location.

While no one was looking (as is my usual modus operandi), I grabbed three bags and quickly retreated to my office.

I opened Bag #1 and emptied the contents onto a paper towel. There were six M & M's!

Honestly, this was the first time I had ever counted.

I opened Bag #2; there were seven.

Bag #3 had eight!

No kidding!

I consumed all 21 quickly.

I couldn't help but ponder the following:

Would a fourth bag have had five, nine or one of the previously mentioned amounts?

I'll let you know of any added research on this topic in the future.

It was a sobering reminder that not all fun bags are created equal.

Why did I get home so late today?

A 60-year-old man with a history of hepatitis C, cirrhosis, hypertension, diabetes, peripheral vascular disease, renal impairment, degenerative joint disease, previous stroke, and previous below the knee amputation, "dropped by" the office today in the middle of a hectic day.

Patient: "My daughter (who has been his caregiver for a number of years) is getting married this Saturday (two days from now) and will be moving out of the house on Sunday (three days from now). She does all my cooking, cleaning, and makes sure I take all my medications on time. I need for you to get me into an assisted living facility tomorrow."

Oh yeah, that's why I got home late today.

Work Zzzz's.

A 41-year-old man was upset because he was fired from his job working for a security company. He worked the graveyard shift at a rental complex.

Me: Why were you fired?

Patient: Because my boss found me sleeping on the job.

Me: You were the night security guard?

Patient: Yeah, but there wasn't much to watch so it was hard to keep awake.

Me: Didn't they give you a second chance.

Patient: Yeah, they didn't fire me until it happened for the third time.

Me: Are you looking for another job?

Patient: Yeah, I'm hoping to catch on with another company doing the same thing.

Me: You still want to work through the night as a night security guard?

Patient: Yeah, I seem to work best at that time of the day.

He didn't laugh or smile, so I decided to just move on to a more arousing topic.

E.D. and wrinkles.

I've had the most success in getting patients to quit tobacco over the years by offering the following information:

For men--tobacco smoking has been linked to a higher incidence of erectile dysfunction (E.D.). For women--tobacco smoking has been linked to a higher incidence of facial wrinkles.

A discussion about the loss of sexual potency and looking older than others your age who don't smoke seems to create a lot more interest in quitting than reviewing the list of other possible adverse effects of smoking--COPD, multiple cancers, etc., especially in the younger population.

It's not surprising.

Can I tell a fib?

Like most docs, my recommendation for an individual to stop smoking often seems to fall upon a deaf ear.

However, I can't tell you how many times I've seen tears well up in a person's eyes when I tell them a chest X-ray or pulmonary function test shows some early signs of emphysema.

Sometimes, it has re-opened a closed door and allowed discussions concerning quitting to be re-started.

It often makes me think about wanting to tell all smokers the same thing, even when the CXR and PFT's don't show any signs of pulmonary disease yet.

I've also often felt we would have a much healthier society if all overweight folks could be diagnosed with type 2 diabetes.

Most of us go through a good part of our life eating whatever we want, whenever we want and in whatever quantity we want.

A lot of overweight patients seem to want to get serious about dieting and weight loss only after they have been diagnosed with diabetes.

I always let patients know they can be healthier than they've been in years if they are willing to make changes in their lifestyle.

Resilient and motivated folks with diabetes learn the nutritional concepts that all folks should not only be taught, but also master.

Superman's younger brother.

Mr. R. is in great health.

He's 88-years-old, runs, lifts weights, works part time at a health club and is a volunteer track and field official for high school and college meets.

I saw him the other day.

Me: Have you been up to anything new lately?

Patient: Not really, my younger brother was just here from New York for a visit. It was sad. I hadn't seen him for about two years, and he's really let himself go. I told him so.

Me: What's going on?

Patient: I don't really know. He doesn't really give me details on his medical problems, but he has poor hearing, trouble with his eyes, walks with a cane and says he wears diapers due to some occasional urine leakage.

Me: How old is he?

Patient: He's 83, 5 years younger than me.

Me: Well, you probably just need to give him a break. You're in amazing health for someone 88 years old. The description of your brother describes many of the 83-year-old patients I see. You're a tough act to follow.

He nodded but I don't think he completely agreed with me.

Not a great start to the week.

Mr. M. has been a challenging patient over the years.

He has cirrhosis, is awaiting a liver transplant and has chronic pain due to advanced degenerative joint disease.

He has been on intermittent opioids for pain after trials of other medications were not successful.

His son has been his caregiver.

I was always very impressed by his son.

He seemed genuinely concerned about his dad and always said all the right things.

I came in today to a fax from the local police department.

His son was caught selling his father's pain medications. There will be a further investigation.

My name is on all the prescription bottles.

I could have saved some time.

A 66-year-old man came in for a new patient visit.

After taking his lengthy history, I stepped out while he undressed for the physical exam.

When I came back in the exam room, I noticed he had a large tattoo on his chest.

On closer inspection it was a list.

On even closer inspection, I noticed it was his medical history.

Allergy: Penicillin

#1. Tonsils 1958

#2. Appendix 1967

#3. Heart bypass X 4: 1988

#4. Repeat bypass X 2: 1991

#5. Gallbladder 1998

Me: I've never seen such an informative tattoo before.

Patient: I figured it would be helpful if I'm ever brought into an emergency room and can't speak.

Me: You've got a point there.

I smile thinking about the response I would get if I started all new patient visits by asking, "before we start, do you happen to have your medical history tattooed anywhere?"

Thanks for the reminder and for your service...

A 61-year-old man came in for an exam and his wife was with him.

When he took off his shirt, he had a tattoo that spanned his entire back.

I was able to get a good look at it while listening to his breath sounds.

The tattoo was a naked woman, standing, with her hands on her hips, wearing high heels.

On the tattoo, over the left breast, there was a tattoo of man's face over top of the Air Force insignia (it was a tattoo on the tattoo).

Under the entire tattoo was the name "Jane."

The tattoo and the tattoo on the tattoo had a remarkable resemblance to the folks with me in the exam room (the patient and his wife).

Me (looking at both): Thanks for reminding me your name is Jane and thanks again for your service in the Air Force.

Both laughed, thus confirming my statement.

A 3-month follow-up surprise.

The nursing note said, "Here for follow-up."

My next patient was a 35-year-old man who was usually followed by a partner who had to leave for a family emergency earlier in the day.

I quickly reviewed his medical record.

He was being followed for hypertension and diabetes, was recently started on a cholesterol lowering medication, and was being brought back for a follow-up appointment.

Cool, I figured, should be straightforward.

I opened the door to the waiting room and called out his name.

A male with a complete cervical halo arose from a chair and walked to me.

Obviously, I was surprised.

After confirming his identity and a quick greeting, I brought him to an exam room and excused myself.

I went back to my office for a more thorough chart review.

He had just been seen three months earlier.

The note from that visit was incredibly complete.

Nowhere did I find mention of a neck injury, cervical halo, phone calls to our office about an accident, consultation notes, etc.

I went back to the exam room and just decided to say, "so, how is everything going?"

Luckily, he was able to fill me in without having to ask any other questions.

He had, since last here, sustained severe chemical burns to the back of his neck and undergone three skin graft procedures. Due to the severity of the burns and location of the grafts, he was placed in the cervical halo to prevent any neck movement to give the grafts the best chance of healing.

Had never seen that before.

Me: You've had quite an interesting three months since you were last here.

Patient: I sure have.

His blood pressure and diabetes were well controlled.

However, I totally forgot about his cholesterol.

Feeling new.

Mr. A. is an 87-year-old man who has a great outlook on life.

I've known him for about 7 years. He has a standard response when asked how he feels.

"Brand new," he always replies.

For several years now he has been followed every 6 months for an abdominal aneurysm. He's had two different opinions from vascular surgeons.

One recommend intervening and the other advised continuing to monitor.

It's caused much discussion over the last few years with the patient, as well as with his extended family members.

For now, he continues to feel comfortable monitoring it.

I noticed yesterday that he was sitting sideways, looking at me with his head turned while we were reviewing his latest study that showed no significant change in the size of the aneurysm.

Me: Why are you sitting sideways?

Patient: I just figured I would point my belly away from you in case my aneurysm ruptures while we're talking.

He laughed first and then so did I.

It was such a hearty laugh that I let him know the aneurysm must still be strong to withstand such pressure.

"I'm brand-new doc, brand new."

A good reminder.

An 84-year-old man just doesn't feel well.

He came to see me for a second opinion.

He was cognitively intact.

He had gone to another physician who did a "boat load" of blood tests and sent him for a total body CT scan. He also had an MRI of his brain. He reports that nothing abnormal was found.

He reports that he then saw a cardiologist who put him through a bunch of tests. Everything turned out fine.

A pulmonologist had him get pulmonary function tests and a sleep study. Both did not show any significant findings.

Me: What are your symptoms again?

Patient: I just don't feel well, I tire easily, I have no energy, no desire to socialize; I even stopped writing which has always been a joy of mine.

Me: It sounds like you might be depressed.

I then went on a discussion of possibly trying an anti-depressant.

I couldn't think of anything else to do that already hadn't been done by the other physicians.

Patient: You know my son has been using a medication that increases serotonin and has been doing great since he started taking it.

On phone follow-up two weeks later, after having started a low dose of an antidepressant, he reported he was starting to feel better.

I've also often made depression a diagnosis of exclusion after ruling out other medical conditions.

Fear of litigation is often used as an excuse for so many tests being done.

It was clear, however, that this man was not a litigious person.

In hindsight, it obvious that depression should have been considered earlier in his medical work-up given his presenting symptoms.

Some generic SSRIs are less than $4 a month.

He had over $15,000 in tests before this possibility was considered.

It's a good reminder to all, including myself!

An expensive palm tree trim.

My mother-in-law called at about 6 am to let us know my brother-in-law was admitted to a local hospital at approximately 2 am for chest pain.

He's 38-years-old and smokes 1 pack a day.

I stopped by the hospital on my way to the office, but he was off having tests done.

The hospitalist who had admitted him had left for the day.

I called during the day, but he was still having tests done.

I finally saw him at about 6 pm.

He had just gotten back to his room.

Every time he would move in bed his chest would hurt.

Me: Did you do anything yesterday to strain yourself?

Brother-in-law: Not that I can remember.

Mother-in-law: Don't you remember, you trimmed the palm tree in the front of the house yesterday.

Me: You did? Did you use a power saw?

Brother-in-law: No, I used a hand saw.

He then imitated the cutting motion and experienced the same chest pain.

Me: Did you tell anyone that?

Brother-in-law: No, they just kept saying that because of my age and since I smoke, they need to make sure my heart is okay.

Shortly after, another hospitalist came by. He reviewed the normal findings from the labs that were done over the course of the day, the serial EKG's, the chest X-ray, the CT angiogram, the echocardiogram, and the nuclear stress test.

When given the added information about the palm tree trimming, he agreed that my brother-in-law probably had irritated an anterior chest wall muscle.

He was advised to take ibuprofen and apply topical heat.

I'll never look at the palm tree outside their house in the same way.

Its last trimming cost about $25,000.

It's a good reminder. A cookbook work-up should never replace a good history.

A little; no, an occasional; no, all day long.

An 81-year-old man was seen last week.

His cardiac exam was abnormal, and an EKG confirmed he was in atrial fibrillation with a heart rate in the 130-140 range.

He was asymptomatic.

Recent labs were normal.

Me: Do you drink alcohol at all?

Patient: A little; only an occasional glass of wine. I don't drink any hard stuff or beer.

Me: Really, that's all?

Patient: That's all.

I decided to control his heart rate with medication and start warfarin as an outpatient.

Additional laboratory studies and an echocardiogram were ordered.

He returned 48 hours later and was doing well with a heart rate in the 80's.

He would be referred for an elective cardioversion once his INR (blood thinning level) was within a therapeutic range for a few weeks.

He returned last evening (3 days after his last visit), as I was about to walk out the door.

His wife was with him.

He was tremulous, shaking and his heart rate was 180-220.

His wife let me know he stopped drinking completely after our last visit 3 days ago.

Me: He mentioned he had an occasional glass of wine.

Wife: Oh no, he buys a 3-liter bottle of blush wine at least every day or two. He drinks all day long. He got worried about his health and decided to completely stop.

Me: Thanks, that helps to explain a lot.

He was now experiencing alcohol withdrawal symptoms, in addition to atrial fibrillation.

He was admitted to the hospital.

I "Oughta."

I met Mr. D. for the first time recently.

He's a widower.

When reviewing his diet, he offered the following information:

"I eat the same thing every day. I have an egg and ham biscuit for breakfast, a salad for lunch and get the Colonel's' chicken pot pie for dinner. The Colonel makes a great chicken pot pie you know. It's packed full of vegetables."

When I acknowledged the pot pie does sound great, he let me know that I "oughta get some."

He's 91-years-old, cognitively, and functionally intact, still drives, denies falls, incontinence and works part time for his church.

You can't argue with the results.

I oughta get some!

Re-programing at the fork.

My 2 PM appointment was a "no-show."

The "no-show" arrived at 5 PM.

Even though the "no-show" allowed me to get back on time seeing my other appointments and walk-ins, I was still annoyed he arrived so late.

He declined to re-schedule when asked by my nurse.

Patient (after I abruptly walked into the exam room): Sorry I was late, but my supervisor wouldn't let me leave on time.

Me: I understand but you could have called to re-schedule.

Patient: No, that's okay. I figured I'd just wait to see you since I had an appointment.

Me: You can ask for a later appointment time in the future if it would work out better for you.

Patient: Oh, I don't need to do that. The 2 o'clock appointment was fine.

Me: You came 3 hours after your appointment time.

Patient: I didn't mind waiting to see you since I had an appointment (he had been waiting 14 minutes).

Me: I'll try to help with whatever acute needs you have then.

Patient: That's great, I have a bunch of things I need to discuss with you.

He either had no idea where I was trying to go with my conversation, or he was doing a great job of pretending not to know. I was at the fork in the road.

Luckily, I opted for the proper, professional response instead of listening to the temporary, evil voice in my head.

Me: Sure thing, let's go over your concerns.

We reviewed his health concerns and had a long discussion about the emotional turmoil he was experiencing with his ex-wife.

I was able to offer some advice.

I'm glad I was able to re-program at the fork.

It turned out to be a great visit.

A frustrating joy.

Mr. J. is a 69-year-old with poorly controlled diabetes.

He has fired two endocrinologists and three diabetes educators.

The most upset I have ever seen him was after seeing the last diabetic educator.

He reported the person was so rude he "just wanted to reach across the desk and punch him!"

I have been his primary care physician for the last 8 years.

The entire time, his A1C has been elevated.

He's well read.

Despite my best attempts, he continues to have his own strongly seated beliefs about how he wants to take care of his diabetes.

His most recent A1C was 10.2!

Amazingly, he does not have retinopathy, nephropathy or neuropathy, and his blood pressure is well controlled.

It's frustrating to have him as my patient.

He's also evangelical, spirit filled, loves life, walks two miles twice a day, doesn't drink or smoke, always verbalizes his thanks to the Lord for his health and always ends visits by thanking me for being his doctor and asking for an update on my family.

It's a joy to have him as my patient.

He's a frustrating joy.

Made my day.

I saw Mr. B., a 64-year-old, for the first time while covering for a partner who was on vacation. He came for medication refills.

Me: I see you have a bag with your pill bottles. What do you take?

Mr. B.: A nerve pill, a blood pressure pill, and a diabetes pill (said with a deeeeeep southern accent).

Me: Now that's a southern accent. Where are you from?

Mr. B.: I've lived here (in Florida) for the last 40 years but I'm from LA....lower Alabama (he then laughed).

I quickly decided that this visit could be a lot more interesting than just a medication refill.

Me: Can you tell me a little more about yourself?

Mr. B.: You bet doc. I'm just a country boy from LA, lower Alabama (he laughs again). When I got drafted, I joined the Army and was a quartermaster in Vietnam. One day in '67 I was working on the laundry and supplies and heard a "whee" sound and the next thing you know my guts were hanging out (puts his hand over his right lower quadrant) and I had a terrible stinging in my left shoulder. I was already on my second tour and only had about a month to go but those wounds got me sent home (he unbuttons his shirt to expose a severely scarred right lower quadrant and a large keloid on his left shoulder). I've still got a lot of the shrapnel inside.

Me: Did you get a Purple Heart?

Mr. B.: Sure did. The commanding officer was good about looking out for us.

Me: How long did it take for you to recover?

Mr. B.: Only about 5 months.

Me: What did you do after that?

Mr. B.: I just worked for one company since I left the Army; a citrus and juicing plant. I've been a supervisor and then became a forklift operator. I retired last year.

Me: Married?

Mr. B.: Yep, 42 years, three children, 7 grandchildren, no greats yet.

Me: How's your wife doing?

Mr. B.: Fine, but she had a little setback having to get her glowbladder (gallbladder) out a few weeks ago.

I was running a little late seeing scheduled patients, as usual, but choose to continue. This "interview" went on for almost 20 minutes.

He had another bout of laughter when he told me about getting his teeth out before he got dentures.

Mr. B.: I had 17 teeth pulled out at the same time. That there dentist said how are you gonna get home. I said what do you mean, I drove here so I'm gonna just drive myself home. A little while later, when at home, my phone rang and that there dentist called me and said are you home? I said what kind of question is that? You called my house and I answered. Doesn't that mean I'm home?

Unfortunately, I needed to get on with my day. I thanked him for his service to his country. I let him know it was a privilege to spend time with him.

Thankfully, I also remembered to refill his medications.

Bet that hurt.

A 50-year-old man had a concern regarding a very, sensitive, private part of his body.

He was embarrassed to show me and even more embarrassed to let me know how it occurred.

After he confided in me, we did laugh together.

He, in fact, did have a significant superficial abrasion on his penis and would benefit from an antibiotic and topical therapy to prevent an infection.

He was advised to encourage his partner to fix the jagged edge of her denture or to just keep it out altogether in the future.

He agreed with my expert medical advice.

Some one-liners from the past week.

An 87-year-old man: I think I'm still doing quite good; I've still got my teeth, no hearing aids, and my mind.

A 53-year-old man, when asked if he still smokes: Not no more so much (he finally admitted to smoking less than five cigarettes a day).

A 36-year-old man, with a BMI of almost 50 (ideal is less than 25), when asked how everything went with his visit to the nutritionist: She basically told me I needed to drink water and eat lettuce and carrots, so I told her this conversation is over because I don't have big ears, a fluffy tail and my name isn't Bugs Bunny.

To shave or not to shave, that is the question.

Lately, it seems that a lot of the younger men who come in for a physical exam have shaved all their pubic hair.

Initially, it surprised me.

Now, I've sort of come to expect it.

Here's some potential reasons I've come across:

1. Religious reasons: all the male nudes on the ceiling of the Sistine Chapel are hairless below the waist.

2. Aesthetic reasons: a cleaner, more contained aesthetic look is in vogue for pubic hair.

3. Cleanliness reasons: the crotch is a focal point for heat, sweat and bacteria.

4. Health reasons: to make sure you don't have a rash or other unwanted critters.

5. Self-esteem reasons: the penis will appear longer due to removing the hair that often goes at least part way up the shaft.

I haven't done a poll to determine the most common reason.

Three balls.

It was a pleasure to meet 74-year-old Mr. R.

He had a 27-year military career.

During the medical history he noted that his only past injury was when he got kicked in the testicles as a teenager.

Mr. R..: Ever since then I've had three balls (one is an organized hematoma). In college my frat brothers always called me quarter dozen (he laughed).

I did some quick math: A quarter of a dozen is three.

Me: How did they ever find out?

Mr. R.: I had a little too much to drink one night and let it slip.

During the review of systems, he also remarked that he was finally ready to be evaluated for hearing aids.

Me: Is it bothering your wife (often it's the spouse that seems to "encourage" men to get hearing aids)?

Mr. R.: No, she has bad hearing also. We just now think each other's name is what (he laughed, as did I).

An attitude adjustment.

Mr. T. is a 65-year-old who seems to really enjoy life.

His hobby is wood working, and he shows his products at different craft shows in our area.

He seemed to be in a particularly good mood when I saw him recently and commented to him about it.

Mr. T.: I just had a great weekend. You should've seen the joy on the face of these two kids when their parents bought a Fort I had made.

Me: How did you make it?

Mr. T.: I had a couple of bags of Popsicle sticks that I wasn't using for anything and decided to try and build a Fort. I didn't have any plans, just started building it. By the time I was finished it was complete with a wall around it, watch towers, walkways and even swinging gates. I went to the dollar store and was able to get some toy soldiers to glue at different spots. It looked great when it was done.

Me: Did you take a picture of it before you sold it?

Mr. T.: No, I should have.

Me: How long did it take to build?

Mr. T.: Just a few days. Almost cut off the end of my fingers a few times with the X-Acto knife. It's a lot harder to cut the Popsicle sticks than you would think by just looking at them.

Me: How much did you sell it for?

Mr. T.: $20. It was my only sale for the day, but it helped to pay for the booth for the weekend.

Me: That's great.

It had been a hectic day and I was in sort of a bad mood before spending time with him. Seeing the joy that he experienced with his $20 sale helped give me a much-needed attitude adjustment.

Guilt free results.

A 63-year-old man was having a problem.

He met his new girlfriend through a dating site, and they had already shared many great weekends.

They hadn't attempted to be intimate until recently.

When they did, he wasn't able to perform.

"It" had never happened to him before.

He wanted a prescription to help maintain an erection.

He reported being attracted to her.

He reported respectful communication.

I finally asked if there was anything else bothering him.

He said she's 53-years-old and she thinks he's 53-years-old.

He lied on the date ap profile and hadn't come clean yet.

He could have passed for 53-years-old.

I told him that.

I let him know he just needed to tell her the truth.

He stopped by three weeks later to briefly talk.

He was able to tell her, and his apology was graciously accepted.

They were still together.

He also let me know that all was back to normal.

He did not a prescription.

What's next?

I follow an elderly man who is brought to appointments by his middle-aged daughter.

She always has had "some work done," by her plastic surgeon, since the last visit. She had a face lift a few years ago.

She then had her neck done since it "looked odd" next to her perfectly smooth face.

She's had the other popular chest enhancements as well.

Most recently she came in wearing post-op boots on both feet.

She had some of her toes straightened.

She has made comments about not being sure what she is going to have done next.

These comments are usually intermixed amongst statements made about her dad's medications being too expensive.

I usually just nod my head.

Spoken (unspoken).

Nurse: Your 8 AM patient is ready to see you now.

Me: That's great (since it's almost 9 AM).

A little later...

Nurse: I just roomed your second 9 AM appointment.

Me: Okay (too bad we don't have more folks to put in the same time slot).

A little later...

Nurse: Are you ready to see your 10 AM appointment?

Me: Sure am (since it's 10:55 AM).

A little later...

Nurse: Doctor ___ had to leave urgently on a family emergency. Can you see his patients for him?

Me: No problem (just let me check to see if my clone is available to help).

A little later...

Nurse: I need you right away in the treatment room; Mr. ___ is complaining of crushing chest pain. He didn't call 911 as he was advised to when he called from home.

Me: I'm coming (so I can do my best impersonation of an ER doc).

Thus starts the beginning of another week seeing patients.

Over the years, I've always just tried to operate under the assumption that most days in the office are going to be controlled chaos.

When it's not, it's a bonus.

Just try to limit your sarcasm (to under your breath, unspoken, comments) and always pack a lunch to eat between seeing scheduled and unscheduled patients.

His good name.

Mike is 52-year-old man who just moved to Florida, from New Jersey, to be closer to his daughter and grandchildren.

He let me know he was going to start a business down here.

He had a heating/air conditioning business up north.

He was studying for the state licensing exam since every state has slightly different rules and regulations.

Me: What are you going to call your company?

Mike: Mike's Heating and Air Conditioning, just like it was up north.

Me: How did you come up with such an original name?

Mike: Oh, I just (he then saw me smiling) ...you're busting my chops aren't you (he then smiled)?

Me: Actually, I can't think of a better name.

Mike: Thanks. You know, I've never had to advertise. I've always had such a good reputation that all my business comes from referrals. I know I'll just need to get my first job down here and then my business will start rolling. My motto has always been "we will make you smile." My customers knew I would always take care of them and always make things right. I'm proud to have my name on my company.

Me: You should be. Thanks.

His Vow.

I've seen Mr. R., a 51-year-old, three times.

The first two visits were for acute problems.

The third was for a full history and physical.

He's always worn all white (a white shirt, white pants, white belt, white socks, and white shoes).

Finally, on our third encounter, I had time to ask the obvious:

Me: I've noticed you always wear all white (I figured he would be impressed by my astute skills of observation).

Mr. R.: Almost ten years ago my daughter was diagnosed with leukemia. I prayed and asked God to cure her. I also vowed to wear white for the rest of my life, for as long as she was still alive. She's still doing well.

Me: That's awesome. Thanks for letting me know.

Just fine the way he is.

Mr. C., a 62-year-old, came in for a physical exam.

When I asked him to drop his underwear so I could finish his exam he stated:

"There ain't much there to check but I've always thought I've had such a good time with what little I've got I don't think I could stand to be any larger."

He laughed and so did I.

Very well stated!

Both socks before shoes?

A 51-year-old man was suffering from depression.

He noted he had gone to see a psychologist recently and declined to ever go back.

He was upset.

He finally filled me in on why.

Patient: He (the psychologist) asked the stupidest questions. I went along with him for the most part but finally got up and left when he wanted to know if I put both socks on before I put on my shoes or if I did one side at a time.

His wife confirmed his statement.

Patient: What did that have to do with me being depressed?

Me: No clue. I would have gotten up and left as well.

He seemed to appreciate my answer.

Of course, I thought about it for the rest of the day. I'm pretty sure I've done it both ways in the past. I'm afraid to ask a psychology colleague what it means!

No more fungus among us.

I hadn't seen Mr. H., a 63-year-old, for months.

He looked great.

He had lost over 50 pounds and mentioned he had a girlfriend for the first time in over 10 years.

Mr. H.: Thanks for helping to get my confidence back.

Me (I had no idea what he was talking about): I'm happy things are going well with you.

Mr. H.: I'm so glad you asked me if I would like to treat the fungus in my fingernails when I saw you last.

Now I remembered. About a year ago, he had come in for a follow-up on his blood pressure. For the first time, I noticed he was sitting with his fingers, of both hands, curled up in a fist. Initially, I thought he was just tense, but when I went to check his pulse, I noticed most of his fingernails had significant onychomycosis (nail fungus). I asked him if he would like treatment for the fungus. He agreed. On follow-up, 6 weeks later, after completing medication, you could see the demarcation beginning between the normal and the abnormal nails growing out. I hadn't seen him since.

Mr. H.: I didn't want to socialize because of my fingernails. I didn't go to church. I felt embarrassed to shake hands. I didn't want to go on a date. I didn't think anything could be done. I've been exercising, eating better and met a great gal.

This encounter made my day!

Now I understood.

Mr. P., a 79-year-old, had always been insistent on having an annual PSA, despite his age and despite previous discussions on PSA testing in the elderly.

The most recent result was slightly high, and the biopsy performed (at his insistence) by the urologist showed a "minute focus of adenocarcinoma (not surprising)." The amount was so small that a Gleason score couldn't be determined.

He wanted to undergo radiation therapy.

He was going to see the radiation oncologist the next week for a consultation.

He came to see me prior.

Me: Have you just thought about watchful waiting (I did not think he needed to aggressively treat his microscopic prostate cancer)?

I then reviewed some of the reasons to not undergo aggressive treatment at his age.

Mr. P.: I just want to get rid of it once and for all.

Me: Do you know anyone who has had prostate cancer?

Mr. P.: My best friend, my buddy for over 50 years, died from it. He and I were retired Army and Civil service workers. We were also hunting and fishing partners. He got diagnosed with prostate cancer and decided not to do anything. He went and bought a casket and paid for his funeral. He died 6 weeks later.

Now I understood. I briefly discussed the fact that his friend most certainly had metastatic cancer at the time of diagnosis, not microscopic as was his prostate cancer, but I let him know I hoped everything would go well with the consultation for possible radiation therapy.

Mr. P.: And thanks for talking to me about this. You gave me some things to think about. At least I know some additional questions to ask before I make my final decision.

Cool, he really was listening.

Tr, not Thr.

A 68-year-old man was annoyed that his blood pressure and cholesterol were above goal.

Mr. M.: I don't understand, I've been exercising 5 to 6 days a week on the threadmill.

Me: It's great you're exercising on the TREADMILL. You should continue.

Mr. M.: I thought exercising on the threadmill would keep me off blood pressure and cholesterol medications.

Me: Exercising on the TREADMILL is a great thing to do but many folks, like you, that do everything correctly, still need to be on medications to help control both.

Mr. M.: But I've really been pushing it on the threadmill.

Me: And you should continue to exercise on the TREADMILL.

Mr. M.: I was hoping to get better results from the threadmill.

You get the picture. We were able to finally move on to a new subject after a few more back and forth threads vs TREADs.

Mine for 6 months.

Mr. R., a 74-year-old, comes to Florida, from up north, every October (and stays for about 6 months).

He's a wonderful man but is also cantankerous (I'm sure he would agree).

I'm his primary care physician while he's here.

He recently called (he'd been back in Florida for three days).

I was out of practice, in terms of how to deal with him since I hadn't seen him for the previous 6 months.

My Nurse: Mr. R. is on the phone and demands to be seen. He says it's an emergency. He also wants you to know he had a bad summer up north. He says he should have never left Florida this year.

Me: Okay, tell him to come right in. I'll be happy to see him.

A little while later...

My Nurse: He doesn't want to come in now, he wants to come tomorrow.

It obviously wasn't an emergency (now I'm starting to remember).

Me: OK, tell him to get here as early as possible so I can see him before other scheduled patients arrive.

A little later...

My Nurse: He doesn't want to come early in the morning. He says he's not an early morning person and he told you that last year.

He's right, I do remember him telling me that last year.

Me: Okay, tell him to come sometime during the day and I'll see him between patients with scheduled appointments.

A little later...

My Nurse: He says he won't come and just wait. He's afraid he'll catch something and get sick from all the other patients in the waiting room.

I'm now at full recall...he wants to be seen only when he wants to be seen...how could I have forgotten?

Me: Okay, tell him to come at "lunch" when no other patients are scheduled.

That's what I did last year, and it seemed to work.

A little later...

My Nurse: He says okay but feels bad you never get to eat lunch.

Me: Yeah, I'm sure he does.

Only about 5 and 1/2 more months until he heads back north!

Frequent flyer.

Mr. T., an 81-year-old, comes to our office, unscheduled, approximately 2 times a week.

He navigates the public bus system to get here. He ambulates with the assist of a cane only.

He has all our contact numbers to call for triage advice but always chooses to just come in. We have had family conferences to try and address.

He's cognitively intact.

He's completely compliant with his medications and lives with his two sons.

He'll come in for colds, transient or fleeting headaches, skin tears, a splinter in his finger, an isolated, slightly elevated home blood pressure reading, etc., etc.

Most recently he came in due to a disturbing dream.

I was able to obtain his records from his previous health care facility and this has been his modus operandi for many years.

He usually just needs a brief exam and reassurance and heads home satisfied and thankful.

When my nurse noticed he was in again she said, "Mr. T. hadn't been in for a while. Where has he been?"

My only reply was, "you missed his last two visits because you were on vacation last week for your son's wedding."

Let's see...ah, no.

A 56-year-old man requested "a brief minute of time" in the middle of a hectic day. He didn't have an appointment.

Patient: I just need a quick favor. I need you to write a note that says I was sick last week and that my son stayed home from college for the day to take care of me.

Me: Is everything all right?

Patient: He didn't go in for an exam because he didn't feel he was ready and now the professor is giving him a hard time because it was an unexcused absence. A bad grade will ruin his over-all grade for the semester.

Me: Were you sick?

Patient: No, but could you just do this favor for me?

Me: Ah..., no. Sorry I can't help your son. I would just tell him to tell the professor the truth. There might be additional assignments or projects he can do for extra-credit. Anything else?

Patient: Nope.

He wasn't pleased.

The Unabomber.

Mr. D. is a nice, eccentric, 81-year-old.

He's had a nickname (just amongst my staff), the Unabomber, for the last year.

He carries a briefcase with him everywhere he goes.

Instead of wearing a watch he carries an old-fashioned alarm clock that he has duct taped to the side of the briefcase.

He always arrives very early for his appointments.

Last year he came in for an appointment that was scheduled a few hours after fasting blood work was done.

He placed his briefcase, with the alarm clock duct taped to it, in the corner of our waiting room while he went over to the next building to get something to eat.

He didn't tell any staff members that he had left it there.

Another patient, in the waiting room, noticed it while reading a magazine and, not surprisingly, thought it might be a bomb.

I wasn't initially aware of the commotion taking place in the waiting room.

By the time Mr. D. returned to our office, the police were just about to call in the bomb squad.

Mr. D. felt bad.

He's had his nickname since then.

Words of wisdom.

A 74-year-old man reported some family stress.

A grandson, who was in college, had recently been charged with a DUI and his father (my patients' son) was reportedly beside himself and threatening to take his son out of college.

Me: How are you doing with everything?

Patient: Fine. He's a good kid. He's always been a good kid. He's never gotten into trouble before. I told my son that we should be thankful no one got hurt and I reminded him that both of us have driven after drinking in the past and gotten away with it. He did nothing that we didn't do at his age. He just got caught. I'm sure my grandson has learned his lesson. It's just a real expensive life-lesson.

No approval granted.

A 44-year-old woman wanted an approval on an herbal supplement that she was interested in taking to improve her "cardiovascular health and energy."

I'm usually open to folks trying supplements if I can recognize some of the ingredients.

I didn't recognize any this time.

She repeatedly pointed out the heading at the top that said, "PROVIDED BY NATURE, PROVEN BY SCIENCE."

I pointed out the disclaimer at the bottom of the page:

THIS PRODUCT IS NOT INTENDED TO DIAGNOSIS, TREAT, CURE OR PREVENT ANY DISEASE PROCESS.
I wouldn't give my approval until I could research the supplement in greater detail.

I don't think she cared about my opinion.

She noted she had already purchased it through the mail and was already taking it.

Two attempts trying to quit cigarettes.

#1. The pastor of our church let us know he tried to quit smoking while in Seminary school in Ohio. He spent many weekends, while in school, filling in for pastors in various parts of the state who were away on vacation. He reports driving down the highway on his way to preach while asking God to take away his urge to smoke. He would crumple up the pack in his possession and throw it out the window of the car. A short time later he would stop at a convenience store to buy a new pack. He reports there were partially full cigarette packs all over the highways of Ohio for a couple of years.

#2. My father-in-law reports that the last time he quit for three weeks he was just looking for an excuse to start again. He was hoping, looking for something to use as an excuse. He started to hope that an appliance would break, the roof would leak, anything. For three weeks nothing happened. Finally, he and my mother-in-law were going to go out to dinner together. He wanted to wear his favorite shirt and it was dirty. He was irritated and therefore used this reason as his excuse to re-start.

An impressive specimen.

Mr. S. is an amazingly spry 87-year-old.

He's not on medications, is cognitively intact, walks unaided and is still the lead vocalist for an oldies band.

My nurse recently placed a sticky note on his chart for me to see before I went into the exam room.

It stated, "87 y/o, WOW!"

Me (on entering the exam room): My nurse is impressed by you. Look at this note she put on your chart. Before we start, I need to know, did she try and flirt with you?

Mr. S.: Oh no, …I'm still the one who chases the girls…I just can't catch them anymore (he laughed).

Me: Do you have a significant other currently?

Mr. S.: You bet. I stopped looking for a much younger women cause they're looking for the same thing I'm looking for…money (he laughed again). I have a nice companion for the last few years, and I guess she is a young thing…only 73 years old.

His only assignment.

A 26-year-old man recently came in for his first visit.

He was 6 foot and weighed exactly 300 pounds.

He was married, had 4 daughters and a fifth on the way.

He worked and they were living with his in-laws to save up money to try and buy their first home.

He reported that he and his wife had a great relationship and that they got along great with his in-laws.

He medically retired from the military one and 1/2 years ago, when he weighed 223 pounds, due to knee problems.

He had gained 77 pounds in approximately 18 months!

I let him know I would do everything possible to help him.

I decided to keep things simple to start.

His only assignment until the next appointment was as follows:

#1. Buy a scale.

#2. Do not gain any more weight.

Sure...I'll try to help.

A man and his wife came in for an unscheduled visit.

They had a request.

The patient wanted me to write him a letter that stated he moved to Florida for health reasons after a heart bypass and that his wife resigned her job to accompany him to Florida. She was trying to claim unemployment benefits from the state they moved from.

When I inquired about having his physician up north write the letter, I was informed that the physician left his previous practice, and no one knew how to get in touch with him (maybe he moved to Florida also?).

When I inquired what "health reasons" were given for the reason for moving he let me know that he could exercise more due to the warmer weather and avoid the harsh winter climates (I guess I'll buy that).

The wife reported she wasn't going to claim unemployment benefits, but she had no idea it would be so tough to find a job down here (I guess they didn't read the newspaper before moving about the record unemployment rates in Florida. Also, another good reminder--don't quit/resign a job until you have another already lined up).

They were courteous and not demanding in their demeanor (which was a nice change).

I therefore wrote a very quick note along the lines of:

He was advised to move to Florida, by his former physician, to assist with his rehabilitation after his heart bypass and his wife therefore resigned her job to accompany him. Her presence here is helpful to assist in his emotional well-being and with some IADLs (Instrumental activities of daily living).

I'm not sure the unemployment bureau will accept the note, but it was about the best I could do with the information gathered.

They seemingly left happy.

A thanks flashback.

I recently forgot about a patient in my waiting room.

A staff member let me know at about 1 PM, when I was about to walk into a room to see another patient, that he had come in to pick up a parking disability form I had filled out for him.

I said, "I'll bring it out to the waiting room shortly."

I forgot.

At about 5 PM a different staff member let me know the same patient had gone up to the desk to inquire about his form.

He had been patiently sitting all afternoon.

I walked the form to him and apologized for the wait.

Surprisingly, he just said, "thanks."

I had a flashback.

During residency, while doing an ER rotation, a fellow resident, who was going off duty, signed a patient out to me in bed #12 at approximately 11 PM (it was a 25-bed emergency room). A blood test was pending and if his blood count was okay, he could be discharged home. The curtain was pulled. It ended up being a typically busy night. I totally forgot about the poor fellow in bed #12. During check out rounds at 7 AM, the attending wanted to know what was going on in bed #12.

Yikes!

I let him know I was on top of it.

I reviewed the labs that had returned at 11:20 PM, woke the nice man up, let him know his labs were fine and that he could go home.

Surprisingly he just said, "thanks."

Similar thoughts and words.

An 89-year-old man lives in an assisted living facility (ALF).

Me: How's the food?

Patient: Great; you know I would never complain about any food made for me, prepared by someone's efforts. I'm just real thankful.

Me: You and I think a lot alike (and we even talk alike...see below).

My wife is a great cook and I love to eat. She used to make tuna casserole every so often. I hate tuna casserole, but I never told my wife. I love tuna sandwiches and tuna melts but have always despised tuna casserole. Finally, one day my wife said, "you don't like tuna casserole, do you?" "Why do you ask?" "Because you never have seconds, and you have seconds on everything else I make." "You're right, I hate tuna casserole." "Why didn't you tell me?" "Because I would never complain about any food made for me, by you. I'm just real thankful for everything you do."

We haven't had tuna casserole since.

Verbal vs visual.

A 39-year-old man reported 10/10 chronic pain and to being miserable and unable to work or hold down a job.

He had already applied for disability.

He was impeccably dressed and well-groomed with perfect teeth, hair, eyebrows, polished fingernails and wore an assortment of gold bling (earrings, necklaces, rings, and a huge watch).

I decided to not mention that his appearance was not consistent with his reported level of pain or his inability to work.

A whole lot of suing going on...

A local malpractice attorney runs an ad on a local radio show every day.

Unfortunately, I always hear it on my way to work, while trying to listen to sports radio.

The attorney, in the ad, notes that he believes most doctors are good but states that over 90% of malpractice is committed by less than 10% of physicians.

Recently, I read one of my medical newspapers.

The headline stated, "Study: Most Doctors Face A Malpractice Claim by age 65."

In low-risk specialties (family medicine, pediatrics, psychiatry), 36% of physicians were projected to face their first claim by age 45 and 75% by age 65.

In high-risk specialties (neurosurgery, general surgery, OB/GYN), an estimated 88% were projected to face their first claim by age 45 and 99% by age 65.

A staggering 19% of neurosurgeons face a claim EVERY year!

While many claims do not result in a payment to the patient, they still involve significant monetary costs to both the physician and the insurer and results in loss of productivity because the physician often needs to cut back on patient care due to everything involved with the lawsuit.

I haven't mentioned the emotional effect of being named in a suit (all who have been sued will know exactly what I'm talking about). There's a whole lot of suing going on.

Family, where art thou?

I recently made a home visit to see Mr. D., a 92-year-old retiree, who is also a WWII Veteran. I was meeting him for the first time.

In the war he participated in the 1st wave of C-47's that brought the wounded from Omaha beach to the inland hospitals.

He lives alone since his wife of 71 years (his high-school sweetheart) has severe Alzheimer's dementia and has been residing in a Nursing Home for the last year. He visits her as frequently as possible.

His home was full of framed and unframed family pictures.

Mr. D.'s health, physically and cognitively, is failing.

He wishes to remain home for as long as possible (he would prefer to stay at his home until his death).

He has all the help that he agrees to accept (and pay for).

Like most families, I'm sure there are many unique family issues/dynamics below the surface. It was great to spend time with him.

On the drive back to the office, however, I couldn't stop thinking about the song "You don't bring me flowers anymore."

It would be awesome if, somehow, one of his family members (4 children and 9 grandchildren) could live with him, at his home, during whatever time he has left.

Flea market weekends.

I have a lot of patients who have a spot at a flea-market every weekend.

Most pay $8-$12/day, depending on the day and the location.

Most, it seems, don't care if they make any money (although they do prefer to at least break even).

One elderly man who sells knives explained the reason. "It gets me out of the house, I've got some good buds there and it gives me and my wife some time away from each other, which we both need!"

If I only knew...

I had the pleasure of meeting a 96-year-old man and his 94-year-old wife recently.

They still (with the help of a home care agency) lived in their home.

After reviewing his past medical history, he stated, "if I knew I was going to live this long I would have taken better care of myself when I was younger."

We all laughed.

A positive spin...I like it!

An 80-year-old man (who had been married for the last 58 years) made the following statement:

"My wife and I haven't had sex for the last 18 years because of her stroke (she still has significant residual disabilities) and because God stopped giving me the ability for my penis to get hard at about the same time. We're fine and thankful to be alive and to still have each other."

That was a great way to look at an issue that is often so troublesome for so many others.

A great reminder.

I made a home visit to see Mr. I.

He is a very frail 80-year-old with end stage Parkinson's disease, a previous stroke, is unable to swallow, has unintelligible speech, multiple joint contractures, and early-stage pressure injuries.

His wife and I had a wonderful conversation (she's 78 years old).

Before I left, she asked if she could show me some family pictures. Seeing Mr. I. when he was a distinguished looking, burly, younger family man and full of life was an honor and a privilege...and a great reminder of the wonderful times they shared in their life together.

2 chairs separated by a table.

Most every home I've been to, while making visits, in which the spouses are still living, seems to have a common furniture arrangement, in whatever room they use as a den.

Do you remember the show "*All in the Family* (the main characters were Archie and Edith)?"

They all have an Archie and an Edith chair in front of a large TV, separated by a small table that has a potpourri of stuff (opened and unopened mail, magazines, TV remotes, pill bottles, medication organizers, etc.).

One evening recently I informed my wife about my astute observational skills (in terms of noticing the furniture arrangement).

"It's funny how many people have an Archie and Edith chair," I said.

She then walked me out into our living room (that serves as our den) and pointed to our furniture arrangement.

"Oh yeah, you're right, we do too...thanks Edith."

Fill a void.

A 71-year-old man: I need you to refill my cholesterol and blood pressure medication and then also throw in a little Sildenafil (Brand name Viagra) as well, will ya?

Me: Have you taken Sildenafil before?

Patient: No, but I just met a real nice lady whose husband died a few years ago and she says she wants me to fill a void in her life. I'm hoping the Sildenafil will allow me to do just that.

A 1943 version of a match service.

I met Mr. R. recently.

He's an 88-year-old that lives with his wife of 66 years (she's 84 years old).

Me: How did you meet?

Wife: When I was in high school, we were all asked to write letters to U.S. service men overseas. I wrote to a fellow who was from my hometown. He wrote back thanking me for the letter and let me know one of his buddies was lonely and could also use a letter. I sent a letter to Ron (her husband), he wrote back, and we just kept on writing each other. We got married when he returned. I ran into the boy from my hometown years later and we joked about it. He said, "I told you to write him, not marry him." We've had our ups and downs over the years but in general, have been so blessed.

Now that's an awesome story!

Have enough time?

I spent time with a couple recently who has been married for almost 70 years.

The wife pretty much finishes all her husband's sentences.

Whenever I would him a question, he would seemingly take a moment to scan his memory banks prior to answering.

Then, often after he said just a few words, his wife would interrupt to see how much time I had left to spend with him because she knew a particular answer would take some time.

"Doctor, are you sure you have enough time to hear the whole story...I've been hearing the same stories now for almost 70 years...if you let him keep on talkin', he will just go on and on and on."

If I only knew then what I know now.

An 82-year-old man made the following statement:

"I look back on my life and ask what really happened? There are a lot of things I would have done differently, but I'm not sure what I could have possibly changed given all my life circumstances."

I let him know we have all probably had similar thoughts over the years and was then able to re-direct him by letting him talk about all his many successes over his life (being a husband, father, having a successful business career, etc.).

We both felt better after that.

A short military career, unfortunately.

A middle-aged man came in with a "high and tight haircut" and was wearing a U.S. Marine Corps shirt.

I asked, "What years active duty?"

Patient: 1977.

Me: How long were you in?

Patient: I was medically discharged.

Me: What happened?

Patient: I hurt my right shoulder on the 4th day of bootcamp doing PT (physical training). I got medically discharged on the 9th day.

I know he would have preferred to have had a much longer military career.

I will not ask him the same question again.

His angel.

Met 69-year-old Mr. M. recently.

He has a rapidly progressive form of multiple sclerosis.

His ex-wife is his 24/7 caregiver. They were married for 35 years and had two children together.

He strayed from the marriage, eventually divorced her, and got remarried to another woman.

The other woman left him soon after his multiple sclerosis was diagnosed. They were married for less than one year.

He was alone and his disease progressed quickly despite all attempts at inducing remission.

His ex-wife offered to care for him. He accepted.

She does get some assistance through a home health agency but otherwise meets all his caregiving needs.

She sleeps in a recliner next to his specialized hospital bed every night. She's a loving, forgiving person.

The tough.

When the going gets tough... ...the tough get going.

1. Mrs. G. was married for only 2 months to Mr. G. (a second marriage for both), when (50-year-old) Mr. G. underwent emergency open heart surgery. The operation was complicated by hypoxia. Mr. G. is now in a persistent vegetative state. Mrs. G. remains completely devoted to him and is his 24/7 caregiver.

2. Mrs. H. was married for only two years to Mr. H. (a second marriage for both), when (78-year-old) Mr. H. was found to have a rapidly progressing form of dementia. Mrs. H. remains completely devoted to him and is his 24/7 caregiver.

When faced with very difficult situations, to men they had been married to for only a short time, both women have assumed a role that many others would not have chosen to perform.

Some may have even "walked away."

Infomercial influence.

I met Mr. B. and his wife. He's a 74-year-old who had a stroke and has significant right sided weakness and a very unsteady gait.

His wife is also quite frail.

As we talked, I couldn't help but notice, in the den of their home, many exercise products I had seen on infomercials over the years.

There was also a large unopened box up against the wall. I asked about it.

The wife let me know it was "*The Total Gym.*"

They were waiting for their daughter to come help set it up for them. We had a long discussion.

Even though it's an excellent piece of equipment, I let them know it would be quite a while before he could safely obtain any meaningful benefit from it.

I also let them know I would have a physical therapist come to their home as soon as possible to help devise a home exercise program.

They asked if I would write a letter for them to help get a refund. I let them know I would.

Unfortunately, I couldn't do the same for the six other open, unused, "as seen on TV" exercise items scattered about the room.

I suspect a lot of other elderly folks have many of these same items in their homes.

His co-pilot through life.

Mr. S had a thirty-year career in the Air Force and flew over 650 combat missions!

He was stationed, with his wife and children, at multiple locations around the world during his career.

Three walls of his den serve as memory walls with plaques, pictures, awards, ribbons, and other accolades honoring his career.

At the far left, on one of the walls, was a framed Certificate of Appreciation (COA) to his wife.

It really caught my eye, even though it was just a sheet of paper in a simple black frame.

"In recognition of your support and cooperation in furthering the dedication, commitment and career of your spouse with the U.S. Air Force."

She was proud her COA occupied this spot on the wall, and I think she was happy I stopped to acknowledge it.

Initially it didn't seem that the COA was "adequate" but soon after I could tell that she felt as if all the awards for her husband were partly hers as well.

Very cool.

The Anzio Beachhead.

Mr. H. is a 91-year-old who has some dementia but still has full recall of his 4 months (22 January-24 May 1944), at age 23, serving in the Allied (British and American) VI Corps, during the Anzio Beachhead (Italian beach) Campaign.

His wife had mentioned he was part the Anzio Beachhead invasion. I let him know I couldn't recall anything about it.

He gave me a brief history lesson.

"We (The Allied forces) were pinned down and contained within the beachhead by the Germans and basically unable to conduct any sort of offensive action for four months before we broke out on May 24th to join and become the left flank of the Fifth Army."

I thanked Mr. H. for the history lesson.

Further research: "During the Anzio campaign the Allied VI Corps suffered almost 30,000 combat casualties. While the campaign was controversial, it did accomplish several goals. The mere presence of the Allied force behind the German main line of resistance, close to Rome, represented a constant threat that the Germans couldn't ignore. The beachhead helped to be a steady drain on scarce German troops, equipment and resources that couldn't be moved to reinforce other locations."

The Normandy invasion, of course, occurred on June 6, 1944.

He was another member of the greatest generation.

Further questions?

A 47-year-old woman reported a long career in the Army.

Me: What did you do when you left the military?

Patient: I packed up my stuff and left.

Me: Oh...okay, thanks.

I got a chuckle thinking about what she would have said if I had asked, "what did you do when you got out of bed this morning? She might have said, "I pushed the covers off and stood up."

A trach and an eraser board.

Dr. B., a 67-year-old retired anesthesiologist and a patient of mine for many years, presented with shortness of breath and a smothering sensation.

He was found, after an extensive evaluation, to have an inoperable hemangioma that encircled and partially occluded his trachea.

He had a tracheotomy performed and now has a trach tube in place to keep (stent) the airway open. There are no other surgical or treatment options. He will need to keep it in for the rest of his life.

He spent a good deal of his adult life intubating patients for operative procedures.

The irony is not lost on him.

He was able to tell me such by writing on the eraser board that he now carries with him everywhere.

Balance alternative, traditional medicine.

(Initially published as a "My Word" column for the Orlando Sentinel Feb 6th, 2003--my views haven't changed too much since then.)

Most people "into" alternative therapies are not aimlessly looking for the fountain of youth. They're just investigating ways to enhance their health. As a family physician, I try to do the same with traditional medicine.

However, many people prefer alternative treatments, and it doesn't surprise me. Many traditional physicians are not the best of role models in terms of lifestyles, health habits or spirituality. Many of us are so disillusioned with our own career that it's evident in our communication styles. Most of us don't take the time needed to ensure that patients feel they have had a quality visit. Most people are not satisfied with a 15-minute visit that may have been made months in advance, and that, on the day of the appointment, may be over booked with additional patients.

I'm glad when patients of mine feel they obtain benefit from alternative treatments for conditions, such as chronic fatigue syndrome and fibromyalgia, for which traditional medicine has often failed. The alternative treatment community, however, needs to have regulatory guidelines in place that prevent some from making outlandish claims.

Many physicians look down upon former colleagues who have ventured into alternative therapies. I don't.

I haven't met a person going through chelation therapy who wasn't intelligent, motivated, and committed to a healthy lifestyle. I often see people on three inhalers for lung disease who still have cigarettes in their top pocket. Gee, I wonder who will do better. Hmm, whom would I rather work with?

If wearing magnets, drinking Noni juice, or getting chiropractic manipulations enhances people's lives in some way, I'm happy for them. I always ask folks to describe the therapy and to bring in whatever information they have so I can review it.

For example, there's feng shui, the ancient Chinese art of placing things to ensure a harmonious flow. A friend told me about a person who was "cured" of chronic back pain by rearranging her bedroom furniture. Good for her!

Traditional medicine needs to get its act together and recognize the actual or perceived health enhancing benefits of many alternative health treatments. Some in the alternative health community need to clean up their act and stop acting like snake oil salesmen.

The two need to stop bad-mouthing each other. There needs to be better balance.

The new health motto should be "feng shui for everyone."

Tee time?

My 79-year-old mother had cataract surgery on her right eye.

Everything went fine.

She opted to go for a lens that was covered with a standard co-pay, instead of the more expensive lens that could have possibly lowered her chance of needing corrective glasses.

The office staff was putting the hard sell on for going with the more expensive lens.

She's been wearing glasses for much of her adult life, so the thought of having to continue to wear glasses was not a concern.

In the recovery room, the ophthalmologist let her know the operation only took 8 minutes.

Hopefully everything will continue to go well.

Perhaps the surgeon felt my mom would be comforted or impressed by the 8 minutes.

On the contrary, you can bet she will only remember him telling her that if anything goes wrong with her vision in the years ahead.

My advice to all ophthalmologists is to not reveal or brag about your operating speed to your patients.

Most elderly folks would prefer to think you took your time instead of setting a speed record or rushing through the procedure.

Some might wonder if you're rushing to get somewhere, such as the golf course.

You can continue to do it in 8 minutes...just don't tell them.

Shocking church services.

A 64-year-old man had been attending an evangelical church for several years but hadn't attended for the last few months.

At two different services, a few months ago, during an altar call and some "raise the roof" music, his implanted defibrillator had fired.

On both occasions, he was dropped to the floor by the shock, and the rescue squad took him to the local hospital for an evaluation.

He's not sure what to do.

He's had the implanted defibrillator for the last four years and it had never discharged prior to these occasions.

His cardiologist confirmed that the defibrillator is working properly and is calibrated perfectly.

He has some options (stay at home, change churches, leave before the altar call) but he (after some more prayer) will need to decide for himself.

It's easy to understand the emotions that he's dealing with after, basically, being hit twice in the chest with a baseball bat during the most inspirational part of the services.

The dishwasher.

A 56-year-old man was on two oral medications for his diabetes.

His wife wanted to know why he had to take two different medications for the same disease.

I started a long discussion on the mechanism of action of the two medications but quickly determined they were not following what I had to say. I decided to try a different approach.

Me: Do you all have a dishwasher at home?

Wife: Yes.

Me: Does the dishwasher usually get your dishes completely clean if you put them directly into the dishwasher?

Wife: No, not always. We rinse the plates before we put them into the dishwasher.

Me: So, you need to do two things to get your dishes clean, right? Your husband has two medications to control his diabetes. They both help, in different ways, to keep the sugars lower.

Wife: Oh, now I see. That explains it, thanks.

I have no idea why I used a dishwasher for this analogy.

Probably because I've washed a lot of dishes over the years and my wife gets annoyed with me when I try to skip the first step (the rinsing part that is).

For whatever reason, it seemed to work this one time.

A lot can change.

88-year-old Mr. O. and his 90-year-old wife have lived in their beautiful home for the last ten years.

They downsized from a 5000 square foot home to a 3000 square foot home, ten years ago, but now it's "too much house" and they are looking to sell and move to an ALF.

In retrospect, they wish they would have done this ten years ago at age 78 and 80, respectively.

A lot has changed over the last decade.

He is now legally blind.

Her arthritis progressed and she is now significantly functionally impaired.

Finally, their oldest daughter, who was living with them, was diagnosed with a brain tumor two years ago and died recently.

They are saddened by the events but remain incredibly resilient.

They wish, but know they can't, turn back the clock of time.

They urge others to plan as carefully as possible in their later years because "life comes at you fast."

Do as I say...

A 67-year-old usually smokes two packs of cigarettes a day.

I advised he should stop smoking and that I would be glad to assist in any way.

He proceeded to tell me a story.

Patient: A few years ago, I was in a car accident and had a big laceration on my forehead. My shirt was bloody, and the ER folks cut it off. The nurse saw I had cigarettes in my top pocket and scolded me for smoking and said I should quit. The doctor chimed in as well. When I was walking to my car, after the laceration was repaired, I saw the same nurse and doctor outside smoking. I just nodded my head and thanked them for everything. I think they were embarrassed I saw them. I never got my pack back from the shirt they cut off. I've always wondered if they were smoking my cigarettes (he laughs).

The end of some good ol' southern names?

Saw a nice man and his wife recently.

Buford is 88 years old, and Thelma is 87.

You just don't come across a lot of good old southern names like this anymore.

We'll have a lot of Conner's and Ashley's in the future (not that there's anything wrong with that), but probably no Buford's or Thelma's.

But speaking as a dude, I still think it would be cool to grow up being called "Bu."

Quite a character.

Mr. W. died.

He was 86 years old and had Alzheimer's disease.

His visits were always enjoyable.

Despite having moderate dementia, his social graces and long-term memory were relatively intact, and he loved to re-tell stores of his years traveling around the world, with his wife Rubie, while selling insurance for Lloyd's of London.

I had a long relationship with him, so I was fortunate to reside in his long-term memory.

He always let me know it was great to see his "favorite Irish doctor."

(He knew my last name was of Irish origins.)

He would then also always remind me that I was also the only Irish doctor he had ever known, thus making it easy to be his favorite.

He would then always laugh.

I'll sure miss that.

A better perspective.

I was feeling sorry for myself.

I'd been having neuropathic symptoms my left forearm for months.

It's the same arm I had fractured (a non-displaced radial head fracture) years ago.

I saw a patient on the same day, who was considerably younger than me, who needed emergency cardiac bypass surgery last year. The post-operative course was complicated by a cardiac arrest with prolonged hypoxia.

He remains in need of total nursing care. He occasionally grunts, is fed through a gastric tube, and has upper and lower extremity contractures.

After seeing him, I was no longer feeling sorry for myself.

No peach for him.

An elderly male was angry that the wrong "diapers" had been delivered to his home.

He had called a couple of weeks prior requesting to have an order for a three-month supply. He asked for the largest and widest available (he was a big man).

A colleague looked through the list of available offerings and ordered the "XL WMS" for him, thinking it stood for Extra-Large Wide Men's

The XL was for a 200–300-pound individual with a 48–64-inch waist (he met these measurements).

Unfortunately, the WMS was an abbreviation for "Women's."

Almost 300 women's diapers were delivered to his home. There was a picture of a woman on the front of each package as well as an announcement of their "soft peach color."

He was not pleased.

He declined to even try on a pair to see if they might fit.

He let me know he had spent the last 82 years wearing only men's garments and was not about to change!

There was no reason to let him know I really liked peaches!

A few calls were made, and I assured him the problem would be rectified.

A puppy and a home run.

I made a home visit to see Mr. K.

He's a 69-year-old who has metastatic lung cancer.

His wife of over 40 years was there.

They met on the beach in Ft. Lauderdale, Florida.

She was from Sweden and had come over to the States for a vacation with a girlfriend.

She never left.

Me: What kind of pick-up line did you use on her at the beach?

Patient: Man, I was so out of my league. She was, and still is, so beautiful and I didn't look much different than I do now. I never thought I would even get to first base with her, much less hit a home run. But I didn't need a pick-up line because I had a puppy. She loved my puppy and I'm sure that's the only reason she ever agreed to go out with me (his wife shook her head "yes" and laughed).

Small, cluttered, and full of love.

Mr. and Mrs. C. have lived in a very small 2 bedroom, 1 bath house, in the country, for over 40 years.

The home is clean, cluttered, and packed full of memories and photos.

They legally adopted their grandchild, Lisa, when she was an infant because her father (their only son) and her mother were "too stressed at the time to raise a child."

Mr. C. had a stroke in 2007 and sleeps in one bedroom that's equipped with a hospital bed and other equipment.

Lisa has had the other bedroom.

"Where do you sleep?" I asked Mrs. C.

"Oh, you're sitting on my bed."

I was sitting on a small sofa in the common room, the only other room in the house.

Lisa is now 17 years old, a junior in high school, a class officer, on the honor roll and is an accomplished trumpet player in the school band.

She's planning on going to college. She will be the first, in three generations of her family, to go to college.

I let Mr. and Mrs. C. know how great it was that they had raised her.

Mrs. C. just said, "She's been such a blessing to us, and we are so blessed that she's a great kid, not wild like so many others these days...we're so proud of her."

They've made such a great impact, one life at a time.

Lisa's life.

A lifetime memory.

A 90-year-old man:

Before I went off to the war, my girlfriend said, let's spend a night together that we will remember for the rest of our lives.

Well, we did just that, and she got pregnant with our oldest son, and he's been a pain in the ass ever since...so I haven't been able to forget about that night...whenever I look at or speak to him (he's now 72 years old).

An extreme penny pincher.

An 87-year-old man let me know his wife has always been excellent at "squeezing all the copper out of a penny over the years," while describing her frugality. He went on to say, "she would sometimes squeeze so hard that Lincoln would start to cry!"

He was laughing so hard I decided to join him.

Turning a Rock into a pebble.

Mr. D. is a 72-year-old who owned a Bar and Billiards Hall at the end of his street, for almost twenty years.

His nickname is Rock.

I saw pictures of him posing, with a son, at his establishment.

He was the picture of health at age 68, muscular, and weighed over 200 pounds.

About 4 years ago, he was diagnosed with laryngeal cancer and had surgery and extensive radiation therapy.

He was a heavy smoker.

He sold the bar shortly after being diagnosed.

He's considered cured at this time.

Unfortunately, he was left with the inability to swallow and has since been fed through a gastric tube.

He's had many complications due to aspiration pneumonia, skin breakdown and wounds.

He's now frail, chronically ill appearing and weighs about 120 pounds.

Rock said he now feels like a pebble.

Cancer, and the treatment, can often do just that.

No longer question.

I've known Mr. S. for many years.

He's a very ill 67-year-old with multiple serious medical concerns.

When seeing him in the office, I always inwardly questioned how he had such a strong will to live.

He's just been so sick and frail for so long.

I recently made a visit to his home for the first time.

He was sitting comfortably in a recliner in his beautiful, relaxed home, surrounded by his wife, dogs and pictures of his children and grandchildren everywhere you could look.

I no longer question his strong will to live.

Don't tell my wife.

Mr. H. is a 90-year-old who had a cervical spine procedure years ago.

He was having increased neck pain and luckily, I was able to compare new X-rays to others that had been done over the last ten years or so.

In all the X-rays, a screw was missing on the right side at cervical level 7.

Obviously, at the time of the initial surgery, it wasn't needed.

Me: Has any one ever told you that you only have 5 screws, instead of 6, in the stabilization plate (and I showed him the X-rays at the same time)?

Mr. H.: No, I've never been told that...but do me a favor and don't tell my wife. She's said I've had a screw loose for years and I wouldn't want her to know she was right!

He speaks!

Mr. S. stopped talking some time ago.

He was given the diagnosis of selective mutism.

He really wasn't being selective...he hadn't spoken with anyone!

Most recently he seemed to be in discomfort and, clinically, he had a distended bladder. A bladder scan confirmed a significantly over distended bladder.

He declined to answer any questions about being unable to void or if he had an urge to void.

The next thing to do was to insert a foley catheter to collect a urine sample and decompress the bladder.

When he saw the catheter that was about to be inserted, he yelled, "YOU ARE NOT GOING TO PUT THAT SHIT INTO ME!"

It was a miracle!

He spoke!

He then also proceeded to urinate on his own.

One smart rooster.

I made a home visit recently in a very rural part of our state.

I noticed a large rooster, sitting out front, which gave me the once over as I walked by, but just stayed put.

The yard was surrounded by a very low fence.

I asked the owner, Mrs. D., if the rooster had ever tried to escape.

Mrs. D.: He ventured off once, about two years ago, and got the crap beat out of him by one of the neighbor's roosters. He came back all bloodied up. He hasn't left the yard since.

I couldn't help but laugh and so did she.

Lucky number 11.

Mrs. T. is an amazing woman.

She has lived in the same small three bedroom, 1 bath home for almost 50 years. She raised 8 children there, 5 of her own and three grandchildren.

Her husband left shortly after the 5th child was born, "shacked up with another woman," never returned and never assisted financially.

But…he didn't file divorce papers for many years, so officially they were married for 11 years.

She worked multiple jobs over the years to provide for her family.

Her ex-husband went on to be married three additional times, all relatively short marriages (each less than ten years) and died from lung cancer about 4 years ago.

Mrs. T. never re-married.

After her husband died, she was informed by Social Security that she would receive her ex-husbands benefits because they were married for over ten years.

Her monthly benefit increased from approx. $600/month to almost $2000/month.

"Waiting as long as he did to file divorce papers was the best possible thing for me. I'm sure he had no idea. It's the first time in many years that I don't have financial worries. I laugh about it every time I think about it."

More about Mrs. T.

A lot of families need a Mrs. T.

She raised her 5 kids alone (her husband left soon after their 5th child was born) and then also raised three grandchildren when her daughter dropped them off for a visit (at ages 1,2 and 3), and never returned to pick them up.

All 8 children were raised in her small three-bedroom, one bathroom home in the country.

She's proud of her youngest child who's working full time at Home Depot and is close to finishing up her college degree in night school.

She will be the first in many generations to get a college degree.

Her grandchildren and a great grandchild remain the light of her life.

The 9-year-old great grandson sleeps over every Friday night and it's Mrs. T.'s favorite day of the week knowing he'll be there.

Like so many other unsung heroes, she makes the world a better place with her unselfish love.

Too cluttered vs too clean.

I saw Mr. H. today.

He's a 90-year-old widower, who has lived in the same home for many years. It's very cluttered and home to his many cherished memories and photographs from over the years.

He's in poor health but appears to be in great spirits.

With the help of his son, who lives nearby, a home health-aid 5 days/week and amazingly helpful/friendly neighbors, he remains at home and hopes to die there.

I met Mr. S. yesterday.

He's an 87-year-old widower, who has lived in an efficiency apartment at an assisted living facility (ALF) for the last year.

It's a beautiful facility. His one room is very clean and uncluttered and is also home to just two pictures--one of his son and granddaughter and one of his late-wife.

He's in poor health and appears to be depressed.

His son and granddaughter visit very rarely since they dropped him off at the ALF. He's sure he will die in his room.

Would you prefer your final days to be like Mr. H. or like Mr. S.?

I'll take Mr. H.'s clutter any day!

Junior's a senior.

Mr. H., a 90-year-old widower, could not stop talking about what a great son he has.

He sounded so great that I wanted to know more about him.

Mr. H.: Junior has just always been a great son. He's always looked out for his mother and me over the years and I know I couldn't still be living in my home without all the help he has given me...but I also need to remember, he's no spring chicken anymore...he just turned 70 last month.

We both laughed…and I thought of the heading for this entry while still laughing.

He found a way to serve.

Mr. G. is an 89-year-old who, like so many others, desperately wanted to join the Navy as a young man after Pearl Harbor was bombed on December 7th, 1941.

He was turned down initially due to being colorblind.

Finally, a friend told him about a new division of the Navy, the Naval Construction Battalions, which had become operational in June 1942.

He was accepted as a Construction Mechanic and after training at Camp Endicott in Rhode Island, spent close to the next 4 years building bridges, roads, and Quonset huts (used for warehouses, hospitals, and housing) throughout Europe.

He was a Seabee (CB, Construction Battalion).

The earliest Seabees were recruited from the civilian construction trades. Because of the emphasis on experience and skill, rather than physical standards, the average age of Seabees during the early days of the war was 37. The Seabee logo, designed in 1942, by Frank J. Iafrate, has remained in use, unchanged--the Fighting Bee.

It was an honor to meet him, another American hero.

D&D since 1946.

Don and Donna have known each other since being kids, growing up in a small town in Ohio.

Their parents were good friends. They both served in the Navy during WWII.

Don was a Seabee (see last entry), and Donna was in the Hospital Corp.

They got married shortly after the war, in 1946, raised three children and have 4 grandchildren.

Don worked for a metal production company throughout his post-military career.

Donna, in addition to being a homemaker, served as a local hospital volunteer and was the choir director at church.

"She really had an amazing voice," Don let me know, "I always sang in her choir. The only reason I was allowed was because she was my wife!"

I'm sure Donna would have never excluded him; they've been partners for 66 years.

Don is in much better health these days than Donna, but "team D&D" remains strong.

It's a wonderful life!

It's hard to know where to begin to describe my visit with Mr. A.

It's hard to imagine all the things he has seen since being born in 1915.

He grew up in a relatively poor family.

He joined the Navy in 1933 and became a pilot.

He was in Pearl Harbor during the attack.

He flew over 40 missions during WWII.

He met a "cowgirl," Jenny, just before going to Europe and they married on his return in 1947. His oldest son, Bobby, was born the same year.

They had a house built in 1951, one block from a Naval Air Station in Florida, just before he left to fight in the Korean War.

He finally retired from the Navy in 1958, after a 25-year career.

He and Jenny still live in the same home.

They raised their three children there.

Jenny was a nightclub singer before they got married and the photographs from her performing days hang in the living room, as do many of Mr. A.'s military photo's, alongside all the many family photos.

He got into real estate after he retired and although he wanted to sell homes, he just "couldn't stop buying up a lot of places because they were so cheap back then."

The youngest son, Tom, lives next door in one of the homes Mr. A. bought during the 1960s.

Mr. A. is physically frail but cognitively intact.

He takes a bunch of herbal supplements every day and has for many years, many of which are of questionable efficacy.

A colleague, who saw him prior, told him he didn't need to be taking so many supplements.

I offered no recommendations concerning his supplements.

I did make a note of what he was taking to review further and for future reference, if needed...for myself that is!

Mr. A. is a proud American, who had a distinguished military career, has been a faithful husband for 65 years, a loving father/grandfather, and was a successful businessperson in the private sector.

Now that's a wonderful life!

Gloria.

Gloria is the wife of a patient of mine.

Her 66-year-old husband, Mr. B., is quite ill, and has been for many years.

Gloria did not finish high school, but like so many other caregivers, has more than earned her honorary nursing degree.

Gloria keeps their efficiency apartment as clean as possible, handles all the finances, often down to the penny every month, does all the shopping, meal preparation, and laundry, in addition to doing a great job of as caregiver for her husband.

They never had children and have no living relatives in the area.

She sleeps on a small couch every night, so as not to crowd Mr. B.

When I asked how long she has been sleeping there she replied, "Only for a little over four years."

With all the problems in our society that we witness, read, or hear about every day, I always leave an encounter like this feeling uplifted by the personal, unselfish, caring acts, of so many individuals like Gloria.

Not so elementary, my dear Watson.

In my quest to be time efficient, I often jump to conclusions.

When I smell tobacco on a patient or in their surroundings, I'll often just ask, "So how much do you smoke?"
I'm sure patients must be impressed with my detective skills!

Sometimes, I'm wrong with my assumptions.

While seeing Mr. B. in his apartment (on the 12th floor of a housing project for the elderly) recently, I noticed pictures and models of airplanes everywhere, and the Air Force logo on one.

I asked, "What years were you in the Air Force?" (I'm quite the sleuth...aren't I?)

Much to my surprise he stated, "I wasn't in the Air Force, I was in the Navy."

"Oh," I said, "I just noticed all the airplanes and the Air Force insignia."

"Oh yeah, " said Mr. B., "they're all from another veteran who died in this building a few years ago. He was in the Air Force and his son knew I didn't have any decorations in my apartment, so he gave them to me as a gift."

"Oh...that sure was nice," was all I could add, while envisioning my Sherlock Holmes hat being snatched off my head!

Just three weeks shy.

A shell exploded right next to Mr. O., commander of a small Army troop that had engaged the Germans, in Czechoslovakia, on 4/16/1945.

He lost his right arm and both lower legs to amputations in a field hospital.

The war with the Germans ended on 5/8/1945.

Mr. O. is now 91 years old.

After rehabilitation, he went to college, law school and then had a long career serving as legal counsel for a large corporation.

He and his wife raised 4 children, all college graduates, and have 13 grandchildren.

He remains thankful to the doctors, nurses and medics who saved his life on that memorable day, approximately three weeks before the end of the war.

He has accomplished remarkable things with his resiliency, drive, motivation and his trusted left arm and hand.

His life is an inspiration.

Another casualty of the war.

Mr. D. was a relatively young married man when he joined the Air Force during WWII.

His son was 8 months old when he left home to serve.

He was gone for almost three years.

He spent the last part of the war serving as a supply officer on Biak Island.

The Battle of Biak was part of the New Guinea campaign of WWII fought between the United States and the Japanese from May 27th, 1944, when General MacArthur and U.S. troops landed, until the U.S. victory on June 22nd, 1944.
Biak Island served as a vital airfield that was used by U.S. planes to attack the Japanese fleet in the Philippines.

When Mr. D. returned home, his son was almost 4 years and he and his wife had grown apart.

They got a divorce.

It's evident that Mr. D., at age 91, still feels pain from this loss.

Studying Medicine.

Mr. K., a 63-year-old, introduced me to his daughter-in-law.

Mr. K.: She's in medical school.

Me: That's great.

Daughter-in law (wearing scrubs): It's hard but I'm really enjoying it.

Me: Where do you go?

She told me.

It was a local nursing assistant school.

Me: That's great, congratulations, I hope everything will continue to go well.

Mr. K. was correct...she was in a school, studying medicine.

He's obviously very proud of her.

There was absolutely no reason or need to correct his use of the term medical school.

Two J's secret.

James, a 78-year-old man, had a stroke when he was 52 years-old. He has been paralyzed on the left side since.

He loves to "get outside and explore" and for the last ten years has always had his small dog, Jessie, in the basket of his motorized scooter.

His wife has always felt comfortable letting them go and explore around the neighborhood.

Occasionally, she would hear Jessie wildly barking, from a distance, but was never concerned. James and Jessie would often be gone for hours but would always return home safely.

One day, she decided to go for a long walk while they rode alongside in the scooter.

They were about 2 of miles from their home when they ran into a couple who were getting into their car in their driveway.

"Hi, James, hi Jessie," the couple said, "oh, are you, his wife?"

"Yes, I am," she said, "it's nice to meet you."

"Your husband sure has a great dog," one said, "it's great the way Jessie will always bark nonstop, whenever James has fallen, until someone hears and is able to help him back into his scooter."

"Oh, he's never told me he's been falling...thanks for the information."

She said she looked at James and Jessie and noticed guilty expressions on both.

It's good to meet you.

Mr. K is a 63-year-old with severe emphysema.

He has had multiple hospital admissions over the last ten years for this diagnosis and has been followed in an outpatient clinic as well for the same length of time.

I recently met him for the first time.

When I shook his hand, I noticed his 3rd through 5th fingers were in a sustained flexed position; he was unable to extend them.

We reviewed his history in detail.

Finally, I said, "I noticed the trouble you're having with your hand. When did it start?"

Mr. K.: I had pain and the fingers started curling about 9 years ago and for the last seven I haven't been able to straighten them out.

Me: Have you had anyone evaluate them?

Mr. K.: 5 years ago, a doctor said he thought I had arthritis.

Me. Any X-rays?

Mr. K.: No.

When I got back to the office, I looked through all his old records. Over the last ten years, there was no mention of his right hand.

He came in for an x-ray that showed ulnar deviations, joint erosions, and subluxation at the MCP joints of the involved fingers.

Labs returned consistent with rheumatoid arthritis (RA).

Sometimes we all lose sight of the trees (other medical diagnoses) amid the forest (his most significant medical problem--his emphysema).

I usually don't order tests (labs, X-rays) if nothing will be done with the information, but in this case, hopefully we can offer some treatment if/when his RA ever flares-up again.

Really sad.

Mr. F. is a 68-year-old who worked as a cook for the railroad for 36 years after 7 years of active duty in the Army.

He was "on the rail" and away from his wife and 5 kids every Sunday through Thursday. He retired at age 62.

He and Mrs. F. spent many a day planning all the fun things they would do during their retirement, including, finally, traveling together.

A few months after his retirement, while driving to church services on a Wednesday night, he was shot in the head.

The assailant, who was caught and has been in jail since, reported it was a mistake.

Mr. F. was mistaken for someone else.

He survived but he's wheelchair bound, has no use of his right side, only partial use of his left side and talks very infrequently. The few words he speaks are usually always curse words.

They have not been able to travel together.

Mrs. F. reports, "He was a good man, a great provider, a wonderful husband and father. He never used a foul word in his life. He was a church deacon, a leader of men. It hurts so much to see him like this. I know the way he talks now is not him, but it is him...do you know what I mean?"

She was teary eyed. So was I.

The circle dancer.

Mr. and Mrs. M., an 86-year-old man and an 87-year-old woman have been married for 40 years. It's the second marriage for both.

Me: How did you all get together?

Mrs. M.: He was somewhere he shouldn't have been, and I was somewhere I should have been.

Me: What do you mean?

Mrs. M.: It was a dance for singles. I had lost my husband the year before, but he was still married. He was separated from his wife, but still married. I would have never danced with him if I knew he was still married.

Me: He must have been a great dancer.

Mrs. M.: No, he wasn't. He pretty much only danced with one leg, so he tended to go in circles.

Mr. M. heard every word and just smiled and nodded his head in agreement. I'm sure he's heard the same story told a lot of times over the years.

Stepping up to the plate.

Mary is a 57-year-old accomplished ball room dancer and instructor. She never married and doesn't have any children.

She has kept an incredibly busy schedule over the years and has traveled extensively.

4 months ago, she helped to "rescue her parents."

Her dad's dementia progressed to the point that her mom was considering nursing home placement.

He has incontinence and like many folks with advanced dementia, has become loud and bossy, and uses inappropriate language, due to being disinhibited.

She had her parents move in with her.

Her life and daily chores/responsibilities have dramatically changed.

She's committed, however, for the long haul.

"I know you can't really tell it now, but my father was always such a gentleman. It's hard for my mom to understand but not so much for me. Having them here, surrounded by all our family pictures, also helps to remind me what great parents they have been and how lucky I was to have their support in leading such a privileged life. It's the least I can do to pay them back."

Now that's great!

Easily amused.

I often get to travel through some rural areas of Florida when going to visit patients in their homes.

I drove by a motel in Leesburg, Florida yesterday that still advertised "clean, air-conditioned, quiet rooms."

I'm easily amused.

I get a kick out of thinking that someone wanting a dirty, hot, and loud room would have been properly advised to not seek a room at that establishment.

The glue.

Mrs. R. is an incredibly steady and calm woman.

Her husband, Mr. R., is only 57 years-old but his health took a turn for the worse 8 years ago when he was found to have lymphoma and chronic hepatitis C. He had four strokes over the next 3-4 years. He was no longer able to work as a welder. He had also been a volunteer baseball and football coach. She assumed the caregiver role for him, in addition to continuing to hold down a full-time job.

Their oldest son was 17 when Mr. R. became ill. He dropped out of school with 2 weeks remaining in his senior year.

The next oldest, a daughter, was 15 when Mr. R. became ill. She became pregnant and had a child at age 16. The boyfriend's family wanted nothing to do with them. They moved in with Mr. and Mrs. R. Shortly after the baby was born, her boyfriend was the passenger in a bad car accident and is an incomplete paraplegic.

The next oldest, a daughter, was 13 when Mr. R. became ill. She dropped out of high school at age 15 and dabbled in the drug scene.

The youngest, a daughter, was 9 when Mr. R. became ill. She's now 17.

Mrs. R. has been resilient throughout. She understands her husband's health issues had a great impact on their kids. They all made some bad choices along the way, but she made sure "they all knew they were loved and that they always had a home."

Her husband's health is now stable. He walks with assistance; his lymphoma is in remission, and he has had no further strokes on his current medication regimen.

The oldest son has completed his GED and is employed doing golf course maintenance. He's also a scratch handicap golfer and has some folks trying to sponsor him to become a teaching pro.

The next oldest is a devoted caregiver for her boyfriend and 7-year-old child and they recently bought a home. They live only 2 blocks from Mr. and Mrs. R.

The next oldest completed her GED, is working full time as well as going to night school for an associate degree from a local community college. She no longer dabbles in drugs.

The youngest is a junior in high school and on course to graduate next year with her high school degree. She does virtual school at home on her computer.

Things are looking up again for the R. family, thanks to Mrs. R.

A "B" to at least the 6th power.

I had the immense pleasure of spending time yesterday with a 92-year-old man, Mr. C.

His nickname has always been "Buddy Roll."

After serving in WWII, he returned home.

Jobs were very scarce at the time, but he persisted until he landed his first job working in a factory that made brushes.

He married and raised a family and over the ensuing years, became a successful businessperson, acquired a lot of real estate, was a builder (built homes, shopping centers and churches) and enjoyed working as a barber and school bus-driver as well.

He has lived in the same home, that he built, for over 60 years.

All three children graduated from college.

His oldest child, his only son, is still a practicing dentist in the same town, right next to the shopping plaza that Mr. C. has owned for many decades.

His daughter lives on the same street.

His wife died a few years ago.

He chuckled when I pointed out the six Bs in his life ("Buddy," Brush maker, Businessperson, Builder, Barber, Bus driver).

He reminded me of some other things that didn't begin with a B; Sunday school teacher for 70 years, member of the church choir for the same amount of time, and a church deacon for over 40 years.

He's pretty much a local legend.

He has a framed picture shaking hands with then Vice-President Hubert Humphrey, during a visit to his town in the 1960's.

He also had a framed proclamation naming a day in his honor, in 2009, for being a "living legacy of dedication, and an exemplary character as an entrepreneur and a lover of mankind."

He knows he has done "pretty darn well in life," especially growing up during a time of racial tensions and segregation, but he also wanted to remind me that he was "fortunate to live in the greatest county in the world."

Good till the last breath.

Mr. K. is an 88-year-old with advanced dementia.

His 83-year-old wife is his caregiver.

She's in excellent health for her age.

They've been married for 41 years.

It's a second marriage for both.

She's completely devoted to him and wants him to spend his remaining time, with her, at their home.

She would never dream of or consider nursing home placement, though many friends and family have advised her to do just that.

The things she does for him are amazing. She's amazing. I told her so. I remarked that I didn't know how she did it.

She said, "When you've been married before and been mistreated, and finally end up with a good man, you cherish every moment together. I wouldn't have it any other way. He's just a good man."

I hope my wife will be able to say the same about me in my later years!

Slipping off my soapbox.

A 25-year-old woman with low back pain was insistent on having an MRI done.

She had recently re-started to exercise because she had gained some weight since she left the military a few years ago.

She never previously had trouble with back pain.

After an unremarkable physical exam, I spent time reassuring her.

She had mechanical low back pain and did not have any radiating symptoms or other worrisome clinical findings (red flags).

I also spent a fair amount of time talking about the over utilization of MRI's, etc. and the ability to follow conservatively over time.

After some negotiation, we settled on just starting with plain X-rays (she was not pregnant).

I let her know that I predicted the X-rays would be unremarkable and that I would call her with the results.

The X-rays revealed a congenital defect of the lower back.

Although this finding was not the cause of her acute back pain, it was still a call I didn't really enjoy making because she did, in fact, have an abnormal x-ray.

I was really wishing I had not spent so much time on my soapbox!

Just 6 tasty steps.

63-year-old Mr. M. had a stroke about one year ago.

He has made great progress but continues to have trouble swallowing and has had a gastric tube in place for some time now. His last swallow study still revealed small amounts of aspiration, so he has been instructed (by a speech therapist) on the super supraglottic swallow maneuver to improve airway protection during swallowing.

Here are the 6 steps (these are the exact instructions):

1.   Take a deep breath and hold it.

2.   Take a bite of food or sip of liquid.

3.   Bear down while continuing to hold your breath.

4.   Swallow hard with greater effort than usual while continuing to hold your breath and bear down.

5.   Cough right after you swallow.

6.   Breathe

He's been compliant, is doing well, and I give him all the credit in the world.

I'm certain the same instructions would also constitute a pretty good way to lose weight for the general population.

Keep laughing.

I had the pleasure of spending time with 91-year-old Mrs. R. recently.

She's been a widow for over 20 years. She lives alone.

Here are just a few of her statements that made me laugh:

"Does talking to your children bring you joy?"

"No, not really, because they still always just want to borrow money."

"That's a nice recliner you have over there."

(She was sitting in another much smaller recliner.)

"I call it my Bobbie trap chair. Once you get in it, you can't get out. I tried it twice but haven't been in it for the last 7-8 years. Only my company sits in it now."

"That's a great picture of your daughter receiving a diploma up on the wall."

"Thank you, I consider it one of my greatest accomplishments. She's deaf and I had to work like hell to make sure she got a normal high school diploma and not a special-ed diploma. It's opened so many doors for her over the years. I was a real pest and kept pestering the school principal and the school board members to the point that they all knew me by my first name and could recognize my voice on the phone (more laughter)."

"I see in your medical record that you have a hernia."

"Yes, I do...do you want to meet George? He was little George at first but has been big George for the last few years."

"You seem to have a great sense of humor."

"You know I lost it for a while but got it back. Things weren't pleasant for many years of my marriage. My husband smoked and drank too much. We always had an extra bedroom in our home, and it got used a lot."

"Did you sleep there to get away from him?"

"No, he would sleep there whenever I would kick him out of our bedroom...I loved my bed too much to ever leave."

All decisions in life do not have to be complicated.

I've seen the movie "Forrest Gump" many times and, like most folks, have a lot of the lines memorized.

One of my favorite quotes is when he decides to stop running back and forth across the country.

"I'm pretty tired...I think I'll go home now (he had run for 3 years, 2 months, 14 days and 16 hours)."

Mr. B. is 94 years old.

He's been an ex-smoker for about a year.

I asked him, "How were you able to quit?"

I was hoping to get some words of wisdom to share with other patients.

"I was tired of smoking...I decided to stop."

He had smoked 2 packs a day from age 14 to age 93: 79 years!

There was no need for him to add (as Forrest Gump would say), "And that's all I have to say about that."

He was tired of smoking, so he quit--it was that easy.

A small sign that changed a life.

Mrs. R. (the daughter of a patient of mine) drove by a small sign about ten years ago and immediately thought of her niece.

Her niece, Brandi, was 10 at the time and had been unable to play most competitive sports because of severe exercise induced asthma.

The sign announced a summer golf camp for kids at a local golf course.

She called her brother and told him about it, and they got Brandi signed up.

She reported that Brandi had a natural swing and went on to win many junior tournaments, as well as a state high school team championship and a state individual runner-up title.

She had over 30 college scholarship offers.

She just completed her sophomore year of college and was the top-rated golfer for her team.

The small sign and her aunt's thoughtfulness sure opened a sea of opportunity for this young woman.

A dream still within his view.

Mr. L. is 68 years old and was diagnosed with ALS (Lou Gehrig's Disease) and is now end-stage and bed-bound.

He's an amazing man and has a great family (2 children and 5 grandchildren).

He knows that his time left is short.

He retired at age 62, after a 22-year career in the Navy and a 22-year career with the post office.

He was also an amazing carpenter, in his spare time. His family reports that most all the furniture in all their homes was built by him. The furniture was beautiful.

Within weeks of his retirement, his mother-in-law, a recent widow, moved in with him and his wife, due to having advanced Parkinson's disease and remained with them until her death.

He and his wife never considered nursing home placement for her.

Within weeks of his mother-in-law's death, he was diagnosed with ALS.

As I was leaving, I noticed an RV parked alongside their home.

His wife let me know that it was always his dream to travel the country together in an RV.

It was a retirement gift to himself, purchased only weeks prior to his mother-in-law moving in with them.

Family commitments and his health have prevented him from fulfilling this one dream, but he appears incredibly content--he has a wonderful legacy of strength, character, and devotion to family, and he can also see the RV from his bedroom window.

An uplifting exchange.

I've seen many couples in my office, over the years, with very disrespectful communication.

More than once I've witnessed variations of the following exchange:

Wife #1: Tell the Doctor about your problem!

Patient #1: It's alright, everything is fine.

Me (directing a question to the wife): Is there anything you want to discuss?

Wife #1: He can't get it up anymore! It's like a limp noodle! Something has got to be done about it!

Patient #1(with his head down): Yeah, it's been a problem...

That's why the following recent exchange was so nice:

Me: Is everything alright?

Patient #2 (looking at his wife): Can you help explain things to the doctor?

Wife #2: Sure, Honey (looking at her husband and then toward me), his penis seems to have a short attention span lately, especially since he started on that new medication. We are hoping there might be some options to allow things to improve.

With appropriate interventions, patient #2 had an excellent outcome.

The #1's, usually don't have the same success.

I doubt you're surprised.

I'm not either.

Not really expired.

There have been a lot of articles on the question: are expired drugs effective?"

Since 1979, drug manufacturers have been required to stamp an expiration date on their products.

In 1985, due to having a large stockpile of drugs (and facing the possibility of having to discard and replace large quantities of drugs), the Pentagon had the FDA conduct a study.

What they found from the study is that 90% of more than 100 drugs, both prescription and OTC, were perfectly good to use 15 years after the expiration date.

The exceptions noted at that time were tetracycline, nitroglycerin, insulin, and liquid antibiotics.

However, the Pentagon stores its stockpile of medications under controlled temperature, humidity, and light conditions. A medicine cabinet in a bathroom is not an ideal storage environment. The best place to store medications is a cool place, such as the refrigerator.

I would never encourage the use of medications that have expired 15 years ago, but many medications, that have been properly stored, don't need to be discarded immediately after their expiration date.

No disrespect intended.

I saw a man recently who served in the Vietnam War and was active duty from 1966-68.

I made a definite mistake when I asked, "You were a Marine, weren't you?"

He immediately, appropriately, informed me that he was still a Marine. "Once a Marine, always a Marine."

I acknowledged my error, apologized and he accepted it.

It wasn't until I was leaving his home that I also saw a bumper sticker on the car in the driveway that read, "Not as lean, but still as mean."

Vision gone, memories intact.

Mr. R. is an 86-year-old with a remarkable history. He had a 12-year career in the Army from 1944-1956.

When I asked how he choose the Army, he replied, "It was easy. I get sick with high altitudes, don't like being on the water, and don't like staying in one place for too long. The Army was always on the move-I liked that."

He had two children, by two different women, before he got married for the first time. "You know how it is, sometimes you just go walking around and you run into someone-that's how both women got pregnant."

While stationed in Germany he had a relationship with a Fraulein for about a year and a half. "Those were some amazing years. I still smile every time I think about her."

After active duty he owned a portrait studio for many years and then worked as a cook at a local country club.

"It was a rich man's country club but that didn't keep a lot of the women from hitting on me when their husbands weren't looking." He laughed.

He divorced after 26 years of marriage. He does acknowledge that he was to blame. He became legally blind a couple of years ago.

He reported that he loves to socialize, talk, meet new people and to sing Karaoke. I pointed out that maybe he should just go walking around again and see what happens, like he did in his younger days.

He laughed while reminding me that he "would love to go walking around again but then I would have no idea where I was and how to get home because I'm blind."

He laughed again when I acknowledged it was a stupid statement to make on my behalf.

"Thanks for seeing me today and thanks for letting me talk about my past a little...it seems like it was just yesterday."

Going green years ago.

On the way to Mr. C.'s house I drove past a shopping plaza and many other homes in the surrounding neighborhood that were painted the same shade of green.

Mr. C.'s home was the same color.

In addition to owning his home, he let me know he owned the shopping plaza and all the other green homes as rental properties.

At the age of 90, he's a living legend in his neighborhood and a self-made success story.

He worked hard for his money over the years and that's why he thought it was "best to paint all my properties the color of money."

Of course, he then let out a well-deserved laugh.

Fake wieners and bladders for sale.

I perform random urine drug screens on patients who are on chronic narcotics to make sure they are not taking other substances of abuse (marijuana, cocaine, etc.). In preparing a brief talk on urine drug screens, I came across the following statement in an article that discusses patients who are trying to beat the system (to pass the test when they are concerned, they might/would otherwise fail):

"In situations where observed voiding (the sample is obtained while being watched) is mandatory for the urine collection, urinary collection techniques can be quite sophisticated. An artificial penis with an electronic, temperature-controlled urine reservoir can be purchased online."

A quick search revealed the ability to purchase different models online. There's one additional reason for many to sleep better at night...it comes in varying skin colors to make sure it looks authentic while in hand and being observed.

I keep thinking I've heard it all...

Coffee slick.

Mr. W. is 92 years old.

He had over twenty-five years of serving in the Navy and saw combat during WWII and the Korean War. He was still active during the early part of Vietnam but was in an advisory role only.

He said he was a "slick arm" Chief Petty Officer (CPO).

I had not heard of this term prior.

He let me know that he had no hash marks prior to obtaining this high rank for an enlisted man.

A hash mark was received for every 4 years of service in the Navy.

Because the Navy expanded so fast during the WWII years, a few enlisted men achieved the ranking of CPO in a third of the time required by most pre-WWII CPOs.

He let me know that during boot camp he kept seeing the same men walking around drinking coffee all day. When he found out they were CPOs, he quickly decided that he would do everything possible to get to the same rank.

A Navy historical web site confirms everything he said.

He was in the right place at the right time and was obviously qualified to be chosen.

The only drawback, history tells us, was that the slick-arm CPOs tended to be younger and less experienced and many, therefore, felt the prestige of this distinguished position fell somewhat during these times.

Mr. W. was a battle tested veteran when he retired.

He also still loves coffee.

Break-up diamonds.

More from Mr. W., the 92-year-old former Chief Petty Officer (CPO):

Mr. W.: I accumulated quite a collection of diamond rings over the years…fifty-three to be exact.

Me: How did you do that?

Mr. W.: Most of the enlistees looked to me as a father figure. Whenever I would see one of my boys hanging his head I would say, "What's got you so down soldier?" Many times, they would tell me they had just broken up with their fiancée. I would then say, "You got the ring back, didn't you?" A lot would say, "I didn't know I was supposed to get the ring back." I would say, "Hell yeah you should get it back. You should get it back and then sell it for whatever you can get for it." And I would always let them know I would be happy to take it off their hands.

He had over a twenty-five-year career as a CPO, so it works out to about two diamond rings/year.

Same categories decades later.

I came across an interesting article from *The New England Journal of Medicine* from April 20, 1978, by James E. Groves MD.

The title was "*Taking Care of the Hateful Patient*."

The author identified 4 types of patients who might fall into this category:

1. Dependent Clingers
2. Entitled Demanders
3. Manipulative Help-Rejecters
4. Self-destructive Deniers

He went on to emphasize that, at times, a single patient might epitomize more than one of these types.

I was in my first year of college when this was published.

I suspect such categories would not be noted in an article published today.

A looser definition of quit.

75-year-old Mr. O. has advanced Parkinson's disease.

He said he was an ex-smoker.

Me: How old were you when you quit smoking?

Mr. O.: Let's see, how old was I yesterday?

Me: You quit yesterday?

Mr. O.: Sort of. My son-in-law and I quit about 2 months ago, but we've had about 1 or 2 a day since, but none since yesterday. My son-in-law says he completely quit but that only means he quit buying cigarettes-he still bums them off me every day.

His son-in-law, who was in the room, reluctantly confirmed the information and in doing so was busted since his wife, who was also in the room, had no idea.

Have fun and be creative to the very end.

The Three Boxes of Life and How to Get Out of Them is a book published in 1981 by Richard N. Bolles, that reminds us that we don't have to be trapped by the notion that our lives must proceed in the order of school, work, and retirement (and then, of course, death).

One way to avoid being trapped is to take a "sabbatical" from your career and go back to school for a while. Obviously, for many reasons, this is not always possible or practical.

Other probably more attainable ways are to find a way to make your current career more fulfilling and continuing to make inter-generational connections.

"All of us have creative potential, even if it's not the power to produce great music, scientific discoveries, or literature. Our lifetime of experience can give us unique abilities to contribute to the lives of others if we maintain our mental flexibility and avoid getting set in our ways. We can also inspire others by our own personal narratives, the stories of our lives. By showing others that you refuse to be defined or limited by your age, and by sharing your wisdom with the younger generation, you will become an Age Buster. We can all avail ourselves of opportunities to feel we are making a difference, no matter what our age."--Susan Krauss Whitbourne, Ph.D.

Now that's some good stuff!

Looked pretty darn good on the surface.

I went to see Mr. C. today.

He's 80-years-old and lives with his wife in a beautiful, lakeside, senior mobile home park in a rural part of Florida.

All the lawns were perfectly manicured, and the facilities looked great, practically brand new, even though the community was already 17 years old (they were some of the original residents).

After I was there for a while I asked, "This sure seems like a great place to live. How did you find it?"

Mrs. C.: We saw an advertisement announcing a new lakeside senior independent-living retirement community where everyone would be friends, and everyone would be able to help each other. Well, that's a bunch of bunk, I'll tell ya. The reason why all the facilities look so great is because no one ever uses them. It's always too dang hot and were all too dang old. This place is full of old people who need help. When one of us gets sick and needs help the neighbors can't help because they are all old, sick, and already need help as well.

I wanted to ask her how she really felt but luckily decided it wouldn't be the prudent thing to do.

I just made a mental note to cross this place off my list of possible retirement communities.

A perfect arrangement.

Mr. and Mrs. V. are an amazing couple.

They've been married for 62 years.

Both were from Sicily, and it was an arranged marriage.

He came to America when he was 18 and served in the Army until the end of WWII.

He was 23 and she was 15 when they married.

He's now 85 and she's 77.

They raised three children; all are college graduates with careers and families of their own.

Mr. V. was also a successful businessperson.

He now has advanced Alzheimer's disease.

She remains by his side.

"It breaks my heart to see him this way, but we've had a great life together and he's been a great husband and father. I have no regrets over the life we shared together, we were so blessed," she said while gently stroking his hair. Her soft Sicilian accent remained after all their years in this country.

Until well into the late 1950s, most Sicilian marriages were either formally arranged by the parents or permitted only with consent, unless the couple eloped.

The intergenerational relationships of the family were felt to be more valued, initially, than the marital relationship. The whole purpose of a marriage was to have a family. Even if the couple did not love each other at first, a greater understanding between the two would develop, aided by their often similar socioeconomic, religious, political, and cultural backgrounds.

Proponents also felt as if marriages based on just romance were doomed to failure.

The divorce rate was also quite low. Nobody wanted the two families to have a problem. The only choice was to keep the marriage going.

A lot of the traditional Mediterranean marriages were also accompanied by the presence, in the background, of a mistress. Opponents often cite this as an example of the need for attraction and romance in a marital relationship.

I can see both sides of the argument.

Regardless, it's clear that Mr. and Mrs. V. were a perfect match.

A fire angel for the people.

Mr. H. is now 86 years old but appears to be much younger when reminiscing about the old days.

He worked for years as a New York City public fire appraiser representing the people versus the insurance companies for damages sustained to property in a fire.

In general, he worked for commissions--usually 5-10% of the pay-out.

However, he would never take a commission when representing, for example, a single mother trying to raise a family. "It just wouldn't have been right to profit from their loss and money was often so tight in those days."

The appraisers who worked for the insurance companies were always trying to force a settlement of a claim for the least amount possible. Mr. H.'s goal was just the opposite.

He reports he was considered a "hero" to the people but "a thief and a whore" to the insurance companies.

He worked in and around a very tough and street-smart clientele, including the Mob.

He says he got along with most folks well because of two simple life rules:

1. If you cross paths with someone who isn't civil with you, just walk away.

2. You don't have to like people, but if you do the right thing, they will like you.

As an aside, I told him it was interesting that he had never smoked cigarettes.

"Why?" he asked.

"It just surprises me that you never smoked given the nature of your business, the people you worked with, and how prevalent cigarette use was back then."

"Well, I never used a prostitute either, even though I worked around them every day as well."

Touché, I thought, well stated!

No pain for me.

There are many things a physician should never say to a patient.

"This won't hurt at all," is one such statement.

Many physicians seem to overestimate their ability to perform certain procedures painlessly. The fact is, many procedures do hurt, at least a little. I can easily attest to that. I even find having my blood drawn to be objectionable at times.

The recommended terms to use are "this could be a little uncomfortable" or "this will hurt some, but it'll be over before you know it."

I still laugh about a former orthopedic colleague. He would always inform patients that the office procedure he was about to perform "won't hurt me a bit, so don't worry."

It served as a good tension relief, for the few patients who got it, when they could laugh together.

A great gig at the time.

In the late 1940's, Mr. F. was a teenager (he's now 79 years old).

He grew up in Brooklyn, NY.

He would ride his bicycle around town for hours every day. One day he stopped to try and look over a wall that surrounded a mansion.

He was pretty sure it was the home of someone in the Mob.

"Hey kid," yelled a security guard, "come over here."

"I was always a pretty confident kid, and I knew I hadn't done anything wrong," said Mr. F., "so I went on over instead of running away."

"Do me a favor," asked the security guard, "go pick me up a copy of the *Daily News* and the *Daily Mirror* and bring them back. Here's a dollar."

"You know back then both papers only cost 3 cents apiece."

"I brought the papers back and he told me to keep the change. 94 cents! That was a lot of money for a kid back then. Hey mister, I asked the guard, do you want me to bring you the papers tomorrow? For about the next year and a half I made almost 5 dollars a week. I didn't tell any of my friends. They just thought it was always great I had some change and could occasionally buy them a piece of candy."

I owe you.

Carmen is the caregiver for her father, Mr. V., a 92-year-old with advanced dementia.

She lost her husband many years ago due to a heart attack, her mother died 9 years ago, and her daughter, son-in-law and grandson live with her.

Mr. V. is close to total care.

Nobody knows how she does it.

I asked her.

"My Dad was a great father. He was a hard-working man. He worked for years in the steel-mill and later in the insurance business. He was a political activist and was one of the originators of the Puerto Rican Parade Committee of Chicago--a group founded in 1964 by visionary leaders with the mission of better representation for the Hispanic community, and a poet. I always let people know I'm not forced to care for my dad, I choose to care for him. I'm just trying to repay a lifetime of IOUs from his better years, for everything he did for us over the years."

It would be a better world if a lot more folks felt obliged to repay their IOUs.

A pleasant surprise.

I've been to a lot of incredibly beautiful, assisted living facilities in which the residents, I was visiting, spent the whole time complaining about the facility.

Yesterday, I drove to an ALF I had never previously visited.
It seemed old and plain on the outside. The grounds were neat but by no means as glitzy and fancy as most.

Mr. and Mrs. O. (85 and 82 years old) have lived there for over a year.

They could not stop talking about how happy they were.

Here are just a few of their unsolicited comments:

"The staff are always respectful and friendly."

"They always go out of their way to assist and help whenever asked."

"The food is great."

"We could not be happier here."

It sure was a pleasant surprise. It's the old, "You can't judge a book by the cover."

You notice I haven't revealed the name of the facility. I don't want the word to get around in case my wife and I need a spot there in about thirty years!

The Munchies.

Mr. S. is a 64-year-old who has chronic pain and depression and has been on long term pain medication and anti-depressants while living at an ALF.

The staff reported he was doing well lately.

"In what way?" I asked.

"He's more sociable and talkative. He's also snacking all the time on *Little Debbie's*."

I quickly searched my memory and remembered these exact symptoms from directly observing many college friends and acquaintances from the late 1970s.

Sure enough, Mr. S.'s urine drug screen (UDS) was positive for marijuana.

It's good to know my long-term memory is intact but bad for Mr. S. because of the interventions that need to follow regarding his chronic medications once we discuss his UDS results.

A great team.

Mr. O. has advanced Alzheimer's disease.

He and his wife have been together since high school and recently celebrated their 64th wedding anniversary. They moved to an assisted living facility over a year ago.

Mrs. O. reports that he was always a "man's man and loved to take care of me and our family. He took real pride in being a great provider, husband, and father.

"He was upset when we first moved here but I just kept thanking him for finding us such a great final home. Now he seems to think it was his idea all along."

"I tell him he's the boss everyday...I just make all the decisions now. It works for us."

No more room at the Coffee House.

I went to see Mr. D. recently. The home was in a nice neighborhood, but the grass was about two feet high.

A middle-aged woman, who was holding a cup of coffee answered the door.

I said, "Hello, are you with Mr. D?"

"I guess you could say that. He's in the kitchen," she said as she turned around and walked away.

Mr. D. was sitting in his motorized scooter, in the cigarette smoke filled kitchen, with the lights off.

As I was starting to sit down another middle-aged man appeared.

He said "Hey," as he turned on the lights, got a cup of coffee from the coffee maker and walked away.

I could see another middle-aged man sitting on the back porch, presumably drinking coffee.

A short time later another middle-aged woman appeared from a back bedroom. She saw me, did not answer when I said "hello", got a cup of coffee, turned, walked back into her room, and closed the door.

A short time later another younger woman appeared and said "Hey" as she also got a cup of coffee from the coffee maker, put in about 4 tablespoons of sugar and walked away.

"That's my daughter," said Mr. D.

It was all a little strange, but we still had a good visit.

I noticed both the den and the dining room had bunk beds but didn't inquire.

After spending time with Mr. D. and ensuring he was medically stable and safe, I said goodbye and walked to the door.

The first man who had appeared in the kitchen, other than my patient, walked me outside.

"How are you doing?" I asked.

"Hanging in there," he said.

"It seems like you all have a pretty busy household here."

He then proceeded to connect all the dots. "The woman who opened the door is my wife. She's pretty stressed out right now. She and I have owned this house for about 15 years. Things were fine when it was just the two of us. The other woman you saw, who probably didn't talk, is my wife's sister. She had a breakdown a few years ago and she and her husband, the man on the back porch, who hasn't worked for years would have been homeless if they hadn't moved in with us. The younger girl is Mr. D.'s daughter. She's married to my son who's in jail for selling crack. She also has a problem with drugs but seems to be keeping clean lately. They lost their home, so she and their 4 children moved in with us also. The 2 girls sleep in the den and the two boys sleep in the dining room. They started back in school this week. When Mr. D. got sick, he pretty much lost everything and after his wife died of breast cancer, he tried to commit suicide. We told him he could move in with us. It's helped him a lot being around his grand kids. I've just about lost all my savings because I got laid off from my trucking job last year and no one is looking to hire a 56-year-old long distance truck driver with a screwed up back. So, we've got 10 of us living in this house and no one is currently working. When our son gets out of jail next month, we will be back up to eleven."

I thanked him for filling me in and wished him all the best. I couldn't begin to problem solve after such a rapid-fire revelation but will contact a social worker for assistance as soon as I get my thoughts together.

Less than 1%.

"War is an experience that keeps on giving-addiction, divorce and flashbacks."

Suicide rates among our military men/women are at an all-time high.

It's hard for most Americans to imagine many of the things that these young men and women have experienced.

At any given time in the past decade, less than 1 percent of the American population has been on active military duty, compared with 9 percent of Americans who were in uniform during World War II.

"The result is a military far less connected to the rest of society. Typically, when our nation is at war, it's a front-burner issue for the public. But with these post 9/11 wars, the public has been paying less and less attention."

Another reminder: the 24/7 national hot line for ANY service men/women contemplating suicide is 1-800-273-8255 (TALK).

(An easier Suicide & Crisis Lifeline was started in July 2022. One may call, text and chat by simply entering 988.)
Please help to pass the word.

DIAPERS ANYONE?

A drop-down list, in the pharmacy menu, under the title "DIAPERS" exists for health care providers to order different styles of adult absorbent garments/briefs for incontinence.

Most medical professionals have been trained to use alternative terms rather than diapers for the sake of an individual's dignity.

(The most common definition of diaper is an absorbent product worn by a baby)

I asked why such a term was being used in the drop-down menu.

A pharmacist informed me that a lot of hard work went into developing the drop-down menu and that the term "DIAPERS" was felt to be the most inclusive given the assortment of styles and sizes to choose from.

I asked a simple question via e-mail.

If/when you are in the latter stages of your life, living in a nursing home, cognitively intact but frail, and incontinent, which would you prefer?

    A. For a nursing aide to SCREAM down a hall for a co-worker to "bring me ANOTHER DIAPER for (fill in your name) ---he/she just soiled him/herself again!"

OR

    B. For a nursing aide to SCREAM down a hall for a co-worker to "bring me ANOTHER BRIEF for (fill in your name) ---he/she just soiled him/herself again!"

(Even though I would prefer no SCREAMING whatsoever, I'd have to go for choice B every time.)

I haven't heard anything back yet from the pharmacist.

I came across a statement I like from the *Health Guide* (by Jasmine Schmidt): using an alternative term to diapers is "*an important step towards helping the public to perceive incontinence as a medical condition that should be treated with dignity and respect, just as you would with any other disability.*"

Time is money.

Mrs. W. is 95 years old.

She married a younger man 65 years ago. Mr. W. is only 91 years old.

They have had paid nursing aides 14 hours a day, from 8 am until 10 pm, 7 days a week, for the last 4 years.

They also know they are very fortunate because they "only" pay $10/hour.

They found all their help privately, without the use of a managing service/company. Costs would be at least double what they currently pay if they had.

The math is easy to do-$140/day, $980/week, $4200/month.

They also have the other usual expenses--water, electric, lot rent for their manufactured home, food, medications, etc.

Mr. W. reports to being a worry wart.

He really "stresses over finances."

He's worried they will run out of money.

It's a valid concern...they report both sets of their parents lived to be greater than 100 years old.

A full day of activities.

I recently went to see a patient who was living in an assisted living facility.

In many locations, around the facility, they had the weekly activity calendar.

I grabbed one on my way out.

Here's a sampling of just one day's activities (this is from a Tuesday). I added my thoughts:

8 AM: Car Detailing (I wonder if folks without a car can join in?)

9 AM: Blood Pressure Checks in the Activity Room (hopefully they won't be doing another strenuous activity in the activity room at the same time which could raise one's blood pressure)

9:30 AM: Coffee Social (it was good to wait until after the blood pressure checks)

9:45 AM: Aqua Fitness with Mindy--at the pool (good thing they clarified "the pool!")

10:30 AM: Stretch and Flex with Myriam--Dining Room 2 (I guess Mindy is still water-logged)

11 AM: Meeting for Residents with Power Chairs (sort of sounds exclusionary to me! Feel sorry for those without a power chair)

1 PM: Wii Bowling with Myriam (an excellent post-lunch activity)

2 PM: Yahtzee with Myriam (I love Yahtzee!)

2:30 PM: Scrabble with Merry K (can folks who are cognitively impaired bring a dictionary?)

3 PM: Dominoes with Merry K (sounds like fun!)

3:30 PM: Jackpot Bingo with Myriam (1. Myriam's a busy lady! and 2. what's the jackpot?)

4 PM: BYOB (wow, bring your own booze!)

6:15 PM: Bridge (I sort of remember bridge games causing some arguments for my parents and their friends from years ago--->see 7 PM activity)

7 PM: Bible Study (to give thanks for the day and to ask for forgiveness for any arguments that may have occurred during the bridge game)

Man, I'm ready for bed...what about you?

Confession of a narcotic over-prescriber.

I graduated from Medical School in 1985. Here are some of the reasons I was so accepting of narcotic use for the treatment of chronic noncancer pain (CNCP) starting in the late 1990's.

-The World Health Organization developed the 3-step ladder for cancer pain relief in 1986 (over time it became widely used for the treatment of all types of pain).

-A study of 10,000 dying patients published in 1995, in JAMA, in which researchers found that almost half of the patients died in severe pain.

-In 1998, a working group in Congress was established to examine what role the federal government should play in alleviating pain and in other end-of-life issues.

-Position statements by various organizations that usually included a summary statement such as: "Narcotics are underused and have low addiction potential when used for CNCP."

-Numerous CME conferences for catch-up education. No "ceiling dose" for narcotics was emphasized. I remember how impressed I was at one case study in which an elderly woman was taking over 1000 mg of morphine/day, for severe DJD, and remained functional and independent.

-Mini fellowships for the treatment of pain became available. In the early 2000s, a colleague became a "pain specialist" after spending 4 days with a pain team.

-There was little noticeable support for primary care providers in the early days.

-Private pain clinics appeared in abundance. For a while, it seemed as if there were more pain clinics than cash-advance shops or pawn shops around our city.

-Non-steroidal anti-inflammatory (Vioxx, etc.) and acetaminophen (Tylenol) scares.

-Delays in obtaining many complimentary services (PT, pain anesthesia) and the unavailability of many other services (chiropractic, massage, etc.).

So, fast forwarding to now.

A quote by Maya Angelou is very appropriate: *"I did then what I knew how to do; now that I know better, I do better."*

The efforts by various authors/educators have been very helpful, including an article in American Family Physician: Rational Use of Opioids for Management of Chronic Nonterminal Pain.

The efforts by Physicians for Responsible Opioid Prescribing (PROP) are also greatly appreciated.

One member, Jane Ballantyne MD, a pain specialist from Seattle, WA has stated, *"We started on this whole thing because we were on a mission to help people, but the long-term outcomes for many patients are appalling, and it's ending up destroying their lives."*

I now have access to vastly improved pain management services.

As a Primary Care Physician, it feels as if the pain cavalry has finally arrived.

The lucky ones.

Connie is a certified nursing aide who has worked for 95-year-old Mrs. L., 8 hours/day, 6 days a week, for the last 5 years. She does the daily routine for Mrs. L.: bath, exercise intermittently through-out the day, dress for the day, prepares breakfast, lunch, and dinner, oversees medications, runs errands for groceries and to pick up supplies, cleans, does a load or two of laundry, and dresses for bed. She lives in the same housing complex as Mrs. L. Mrs. L. called her after seeing an advertisement Connie had placed in their clubhouse. They agreed on a price of $10/hour 5 years ago. Although Connie knows she has earned a raise, she has never asked for one because she knows Mrs. L. is financially strapped. She also takes a lot of pride in her work and knows Mrs. L. would not be able to stay home without her. She also arranged for a friend to come the one day of the week she's off at the same hourly rate.

Kesha, also a certified nursing aide, has worked for 61-year-old, homebound, Mrs. O., for the last 3 years, 6 days a week, 6-8 hours/day. A "friend of a friend" hooked them up. Kesha refers to Mrs. O. as "Mom." Her daily duties are very similar to those of Connie. They agreed on a price of $10/hour three years ago. Many others have tried to hire her to work for them, but Kesha would never think of leaving "Mom." She arranged for another woman to come in on the one day she isn't there, but only has her do the basics. Kesha is very particular about things like wound care dressings, etc., and only wants to do it herself.

Mrs. R. lives in a retirement community. She's 78 years old and has severe degenerative joint disease. She needs help but can't seem to find anyone she can afford. She has called multiple home health agencies but the lowest price she has been quoted for a nursing aide is $24/hour.

Connie and Kesha don't work for an agency.

The agencies pay their nursing aids about $10-12/hour. They tack on a 50% administrative fee.

That's the part that most folks have trouble paying.

Only a few are lucky enough to have found a Connie or a Kesha.

Double stone plans.

I spent some time recently with Mr. and Mrs. R.

They're both in their 90s and have been married to each other for the last ten years; a second marriage for both.

I asked if they had given any thought to end-of-life issues.

Mrs. R. responded, "You bet, it's all taken care of. My first husband is buried in Kentucky. When he died, we bought a double (head) stone and plot. Mr. R. also has a double stone and plot where his first wife is buried, close by here. Neither of us were expecting to end up married again. We decided when we got married to be buried next to our first spouse. Everything is already paid for. There's no reason to spend any more money than we've already spent."

I wasn't expecting this answer, but it made sense.

The purpose of my question was to inquire about advance directives (living wills, etc.).

It took me a second or two to get my thoughts together to continue with my initially intended discussion.

A white out.

Mr. R. could be described by some as being a "grumpster."

He's 92 and he's got a full head of white hair.

He hit me with a few zingers on one of our most recent visits together.

My favorite was the following:

"You look as old as I do. What can you possibly do to help me at your age? Can't I be seen by a younger doctor?"

I laughed.

He didn't.

I was only 52 at the time, but in his defense, I did already have a full head of white hair!

Day at the Museum.

Mr. M. seems to save everything.

He lives alone.

His three-bedroom home is packed full of stuff.

It's cool to look around and take it all in.

He's only 9 years older than me, so it brings back a lot of memories: different types of clocks, stereos and turn-tables, records, 8-track and cassette players, different types of musical instruments, black and white and console TVs, etc. It's all very well organized.

There's plenty of room to walk around.

I wouldn't use the word "hoarder" to describe it all.

"You sure have a lot of stuff in your home," was all I could think of saying.

"My father, before he died, always said my home was like a museum. I've always bought real good quality things and I've always tried to keep them in real good shape. I'm just not sure what will happen to it all when I die because I don't have any children."

"I'm not sure either but you have a lot of history in your home. There must be collectors or museum curators out there who will really appreciate what you have accumulated here in your home. Your dad was right. Your home is a museum."

Petite Red.

I've crossed paths with some folks named Big Red over the years. All have been tall, burly men with red hair.

I saw Mr. D. in his home recently. He had old, framed pictures scattered around his bedroom.

The first one to capture my attention was a picture of his boat named *Big Red*.

"Big Red," I said out loud.

"I named the boat after my wife (who died a few years ago), " he said.

Honestly, my first thought was that he had been married to a tall, full figured woman with red hair.

I then noticed other pictures around the room of him with a very petite woman whose red hair added about another foot to her height.

I knew I was looking at Big Red.

Her nickname was perfect.

A picture is worth a thousand words.

My daughter has been away since this past Monday.

It seems a lot longer.

It's always sort of sad to meet folks who, for whatever reason, are estranged from their children, often for decades.

I saw Mr. L., a 63-year-old, who has not seen his daughter for over 35 years.

He reports he and his wife had an unpleasant divorce. She had custody and he had visitation rights, but a job forced him to relocate to Florida.

The last few times he saw his kids he felt as if they had turned against him and then days turned into months and months turned into years without any contact.

He had several pictures on a wall in his room at the assisted living facility where he now resides due to having had a stroke.

He informed me they were pictures of his daughter.

He found her on Facebook and luckily her pictures were not blocked, so he could see and copy them.

He got a little teary eyed when he talked about her, but he was also smiling while stating what a beautiful woman she is.

They were nice pictures. Hopefully there will be way for them to re-connect in the future.

Needed: raiders of the lost art.

Mr. K. is 78 years old.

He converted his garage into an art studio years ago and its packed full of his beautiful drawings--pencil and watercolor (many framed, others not).

He lost count of the number years ago.

I would estimate easily a few hundred.

A few years ago, he exhibited many for a month at the local City Hall. Many of the drawings are from sites around his town.

He's a widower. They had no children. He reports no living relatives.

He mentioned that he suspects whoever buys his house, when he dies, will just throw them all away.

He would love for them to be passed on.

I gave him some ideas on how to try and distribute many of his master pieces before he dies.

I hope he will investigate some of the ideas.

I'll have a social worker see him to assist as well.

They belong on walls, not a dumpster.

I don't want to be a foreskin!

90-year-old Mr. H. grew up in a household where a lot of Yiddish was spoken.

We talked about his past, including his very interesting social history.

He has had a wide assortment of experiences and, during our conversation, mentioned he has come across several "schmucks" and "menschen" over the years.

A quick check in a Yiddish dictionary, on my return to the office, allowed me to be more informed.

A mensch is a good person, a person of integrity and honor.

A schmuck is a prick, that portion of one's penis which is cut off during circumcision (the foreskin), a moron, an idiot, an obnoxious, contemptible, or detestable person or one who is stupid or foolish.

I'm sure hoping he won't describe me as being a schmuck if any family members inquire about how our visit went!

A Spiritual snooze.

Amid looking through some hospital records I read a chaplains note that gave me a brief chuckle.

I'm easily amused.

"Stopped by and visited with patient today and said prayers at the bedside together. The patient's theological position was respected, and no effort was made to proselytize. The patient was sleeping soundly for the entire visit."

Here's my interpretation: "Stopped by and visited with a patient who was sleeping today and said prayers at his bedside, along with God. I did not wake the patient to ask his faith, nor did I try to convert him to my faith while he continued to sleep. A good time was had by all."

Where everybody knows your name.

Mr. K. lives at an assisted living facility out in the country, in Tavares, Fl.

It's a beautiful part of Florida and only about 30 miles outside of Orlando.

There's a noticeable difference in all the businesses, however.

In Orlando: 7-11, Publix, Chili's, Outback, Friday's, Denny's, Terminex, Re-Max, Century 21, U-Haul Storage Center, etc.

In Tavares: Jimmy's General Store, Scott's Country Market, Charlie's Grille, Billy's Cafe, Mary's Kountry Kitchen (spelled exactly that way), Shelley's Exterminator and Septic Service, Lou's Realty, Bob's Self Storage, etc.

In Tavares, I always want to go inside and look at name tags to see if I might identify the owner.

I've never had that same urge at the big chain stores in Orlando.

The Golden rule.

Al (Mr. V.) has advanced Parkinson's disease.

Many family members, neighbors, health care professionals and even church friends have advised Mrs. V. to place him in a nursing home.

She politely declines.

"I may not have all the certificates and degrees of a nurse, but nobody can take care of Al like I can take care of Al. I've seen a lot of nursing homes. They do the best job they can under difficult circumstances, but I would never want to live in one, would you? If they're not good enough for me, they're not good enough for Al."

I nodded in agreement.

I could have said "Amen!"

A classic with a nonfunctional convertible top.

Mr. G. is an amazing 86 y/o.

One of his concerns is that he has a phimosis-a condition, in uncircumcised men, where the foreskin cannot be fully retracted over the glans (head) of the penis.

He had seen a urologist who recommended a circumcision.

Mr. G. wasn't so sure.

He had not been sexually active for over 7 years since his wife died.

"What's your understanding of a phimosis?" I asked.

"The way I look at it, my convertible has become a hard-top, but it's a classic. I've just got to decide if I want to have the roof permanently removed," he said with a laugh.

"It's got to be a tough decision for you since you've been riding the same car for the last 86 years." We both laughed. "It's not an emergency. We can discuss it again the next time I see you but let me know if you have any problems before then as well."

He agreed.

His classic remains intact for the time being.

Time efficient Rosary.

Mr. N. has been saying the Rosary every day, he estimates, for the last seventy years.

"How long does it take you to get through it?" I asked.

(I grew up in the Catholic church but couldn't remember.)

"I've got to where I can do it in 26 minutes," he replied.

"Wow," I said, "you sure talk fast."

"I need to. I'm not sure how much time I have left."

We both laughed at that.

Here's some quick math:

26 minutes/day or 9490 minutes/year or 664,300 minutes over the last 70 years.

There are 525,600 minutes in a year, so he has spent 1.26 years of his life saying the Rosary.

He's 86 years old, cognitively intact, and obviously still has a great sense humor.

It appears to be time well spent.

Impressive stacks.

Mr. B. loves stacks.

That's my professional opinion.

I spent time in his apartment the other day.

The stacks were impressive--most were two to four feet in height.

Neat stacks of cleaning supplies, toilet paper, paper towels, VHS tapes, CD's, cassette tapes, records, etc. were all neatly stacked throughout his apartment.

It was a "you need to see it to believe it" encounter.

It was not cluttered; there was plenty of space to maneuver around his apartment.

I couldn't help but wonder the time involved to retrieve, for example, a VHS tape at the bottom of a stack.

(He was watching a VHS movie when I arrived.)

He reports a very orderly way of taking down and then rebuilding the stack affected.

He recognizes it's odd.

Many of us have some minor OCD issues that we deal with daily.

He's a stack man.

Grandi sapori (tastes great)!

Mr. G. is in his late 80's.

He grew up in Rochester, NY.

He reported an aunt and uncle started the Ragu company many years ago in Rochester.

Ragu, by the way, means meat sauce in Italian.

He reported taking bottles to different shops around town on the back of his bicycle and leaving them there on consignment.

When their stock increased, which was mainly dependent on the number of bottles they could obtain, he reported often helping his uncle sell them from the trunk of a car.

It was quite a story with remarkable details.

He is cognitively impaired, however, so I decided to do some fact checking on my return home.

Sure enough, information available on the internet reports "in 1937, on the streets of Rochester, Giovanni and Assunta Cantisano, their son Ralph and relatives started selling their homemade Ragu brand door-to-door."

Mr. G. was 11 years old in 1937.

I'm sure he has had his fair share of amazing Italian food over the years!

Wanting to give a Zoot the boot.

Mr. G.'s history lesson continued.

"I was sort of black-balled in the business industry for a number of years, along with my friends, because I wore a zoot suit."

I just nodded and pretended I knew what he was talking about.

Some quick research after our visit:

1. A zoot suit is a men's suit that became popular in the 1940's, with high-waisted, wide-legged, tight cuffed-pegged trousers, along with a long coat with wide lapels and wide padded shoulders.

2. Due to the amount of material required to make zoot Suits, the U.S. War Production Board said that they wasted materials that should be devoted to the World War II effort. It was considered unpatriotic in wartime and was a factor in the Zoot Suit Riots.

The U.S War Production Board was in operation from 1/16/1942 until it was dissolved in 1945 just after the surrender of Japan. It was given the task of regulating the production of and the use of materials and fuel during WWII.

If they were still in operation today, the U.S War Production Board would be very busy!

Unhappily ever after.

Mr. and Mrs. Z. are both 78 years old.

They have known each other since they were 12 and started dating when they were 14.

They have been married for 60 years. They profess to having disliked each other for years. In passing, they even acknowledge hating each other at times.

Some might ask why they have stayed together this long.

I was one of the "some."

When asked if they had ever considered separating or a divorce, they both stated, almost in unison, "Of course not, we've been this way for years!"

I got to know then better.

They raised 5 children, have "a boat load of grandchildren," and a few great-grandchildren.

Their house has family pictures literally everywhere you looked.

I've crossed paths with many over the years who would have loved to have shared a life like Mr. and Mrs. Z.

A double-take sign.

I saw a patient today at an assisted living facility that was in a rural area.

The sign at the entrance had the following quote under the name of the ALF:

"You deserve the best, but we are the best!"

I decided not to ask any staff about it but pondered the wording on my way back to the office.

I'm sort of certain that the "but" should have been an "and."

Once they realized the error maybe they got a discount on the sign and decided to keep it as is?

Maybe I'm the first person to question the wording since they opened for business in 1997?

Maybe they did it on purpose so folks like me would ponder it awhile and not forget their name?

I'll just ask someone the next time I visit.

Only one out of four.

Mr. R.'s daughter showed me a few pictures from 19 months ago.

It was Mr. R.'s 90th birthday celebration.

He appeared to be the picture of health: socializing, singing, and dancing.

She reported that at the time he was still walking 2.5 miles and doing 200 push-ups a day.

Unfortunately, he fell a month later and sustained a left hip fracture.

A year and a half later, he's still significantly disabled.

Hip fractures are never a good thing in the elderly.

In the elderly, within one year after a hip fracture, 25% have died, 25% remain in a long-term care facility, 25% are home but disabled, and only 25% have returned to their baseline of function.

Only 1 out of every 4-return close to their baseline.

Mr. R. was the picture of health prior to his fall and hip fracture.

Unfortunately, it again confirms the statistics.

Aging and risk for heart disease.

A study conducted in Denmark, by the University of Copenhagen, has linked heart disease to six signs of aging: baldness at the crown of the head, receding hairline at the temples, gray hair, wrinkles, earlobe creases and fatty deposits around the eyes.

The study concluded that the presence of visible signs of aging signaled an increased risk for heart attacks and heart disease.

What a shocker (I'm being sarcastic)!

I haven't done a research study on the topic yet, but it also seems to me, from my experience, that heart disease is also probably associated with cataracts, hearing loss, decreased muscle mass, love handles, arthritis, and erectile dysfunction.

Here's my own conclusion: The older a person is, the greater the risk for heart attacks and heart disease.

So here comes the big question: is it best to allow your doctor to see your visible signs of aging or to undergo hair transplants (for balding and receding hair), dye your hair, and see a dermatologist or plastic surgeon to correct the wrinkles, earlobe creases and fatty deposits?

I wonder if a person who uses Grecian Formula might sue the hair dye company for making it harder for his doctor to consider if he might have heart disease? Maybe a warning will need to be put on the products?

Warning: the use of hair dye might make it harder for your doctor to know if you have heart disease. Use at your own risk. You should notify your doctor, and anyone else you are trying to fool into thinking you are younger than you really are, if you are using a hair dye product.

Walking the talk?

The daughter of a patient of mine said the following:

"We elected the devil, what's wrong with all the people who voted for him, our country is going down the drain."

At the conclusion of our time together I thanked her for everything she was doing for her father. I let her know that many others would not do the same in caring for him at home due to the complexity of his medical condition.

She replied, "It's all in God's hands. In everything I do, and in everything that happens in life, I just always remember that God is in control."

I decided to not revisit her first statement about the devil, but I did ponder it on my drive back to the office.

Mind preservation.

Mrs. N. recently spent some time in a nursing home to rehabilitate after a heart valve replacement. She's 83 years old.

"I sure don't want to spend any more time in a nursing home," she said.

"It's depressing and embarrassing to sit around all day waiting for your 1/2 hour of therapy next to people who have lost their minds. People sitting around saying the same things, holding baby dolls, combing, and stroking the hair on the dolls. It's okay, I guess, if you've already lost your mind when you get there. I was pretty sure I was going to lose mine if I didn't get out of there as soon as possible."

She's back home and still of sound mind.

Wise owl.

Mr. F. is 95 years old.

He is a wealth of information and clearly loves to reminisce.

After serving in the military, he went to a trade school.

He then had a very successful career in the construction business.

He wanted me to know that he had come across "a lot of very smart people over the years who were not very wise."

I decided to just listen and not talk very much during our time together for a couple of reasons:

1. He was quite hearing impaired, so it was easier to listen.

2. He wouldn't have any significant information on me to know if I fell into the smart but not very wise category.

Welcome to the poo.

There was a sign near the front door of the home of Mr. P.

"Welcome to the Zoo."

I could hear dogs barking once I rang the doorbell.

Once inside I met the three border collies, three cats, and periodically ducked as the two cockatiels, who had free rein of the house, flew by.

Mr. P. had a good size spot of bird droppings on the left shoulder of his T-shirt.

It didn't seem to bother him, so I wasn't going to let it bother me.

Mr. P. was happy, in relatively good shape given his assortment of medical problems and all nine inhabitants of the home seemed to get along well together.

I did find a mirror on my return to the office, however, to make sure I was poo free after my visit to the zoo.

Organized to a fault.

95-year-old Mr. F. knows he's a hoarder, but he doesn't like to think in those terms.

He prefers to call it "pride of possessions."

The only furnishings in his one-bedroom apartment are a recliner, one bureau, two desks and a stool (where I sat).

The rest of the apartment is basically floor-to-ceiling home-made shelves with carefully marked and stacked plastic containers with aisles just wide enough to walk through.

I wanted to ask his permission to take a picture, but it would not have done it justice.

He seems to know exactly where everything is located. Even screws are boxed according to length--listed both in inches and millimeters.

I reached for my pen to make notes and realized I had left it in my car. I apologized for forgetting my pen and asked if I could borrow something to write with.

No worries--right next to the recliner that serves as his chair and his bed--were 5 full containers marked 1. Pencils 2. Black ink stick pens 3. Blue ink stick pens 4. Click pens and 5. Felt tip markers.

Each was completely full. I guess he thought I looked like a click pen sort of guy.

1/2 man.

Mr. B. is only 63 years-old, but he remarks that he is half the man that he used to be, and then laughs.

He had bilateral above the knee amputations due to severe peripheral vascular disease during his late 40's.

He kept me laughing during most of our visit together.

He may be half a man, but he appears to have a better outlook on life than many "complete men" I encounter.

I commented that he clearly doesn't seem to sweat the small stuff In life.

In fact, he let me know, he thinks it's weird that he only sweats on the upper half of his body.

He then let out another hearty laugh, and so did I.

Simple pleasures.

Mr. O. is a very ill man with multiple medical problems.

He's been bedbound for a while.

I spent part of our visit trimming his toenails that hadn't been cut in a very long time.

My nurse had given me a heads-up, so I was sure to have heavy-duty nail nippers before going to his home.

There's no chance for a significant improvement for most of his medical problems.

Cutting his toenails, however, sure seemed to make his day.

Seeing how thankful he was to have such a simple thing done made my day as well.

Gold exchange….

Mr. P. is 83 years-old and still has a great sense of humor.

As I was getting ready to leave his home, he wanted to remind me of something:

"You know how everyone says these are supposed to be my golden years. I'm learning quickly that they are only the golden years for the doctors. They get to take all the gold from us old people."

He laughed and so did I. It's sad...but often very true.

Unfortunately, studies do confirm that a significant portion of one's life savings is often spent in the last weeks to months of life--I'm hoping that won't be the case for me.

Good thinkin'.

Mr. M. has advanced dementia.

He was sitting back in a recliner with two 3-year-old Chihuahuas by his side on my arrival--one sitting on his chest and the other between his legs.

I finally asked him their names.

"Come here," said Mr. M.

Before I could ask any further questions, his wife let me know they weren't given "official" names because of his poor memory.

"He just calls them come here. They never leave his side."

"Come here makes perfect sense," I said, "but are they come here 1 and come here 2?"

"No, just come here," confirmed his wife.

I smiled, Mrs. M. chuckled, and Mr. M. sort of laughed.

All (Mr. M., Mrs. M. and the chihuahuas) seemed to be very content.

Old faithful.

Mr. C. let me know that he would never try to be intimate with the woman who sleeps in his bed at night, and helps him throughout the day, because he has never cheated on his wife.

Mrs. C., his wife of over 60 years, is his 24/7 caregiver. As his dementia became more advanced, Mr. C. started to think that

Mrs. C. was just a woman who was there to help him. He's not sure what happened to his wife.

Mrs. C. gets a little teary-eyed talking about it, but she also realizes he was always good to her and never gave her any reason to think he was being unfaithful. She said, "He has more than confirmed that he has always been faithful and a good man."

I agreed.

Quick Math.

Mr. P., an 82-year-old, has insomnia.

"It makes for a long night, doesn't it?"

"It sure does. I try to pass the time by counting all my money and savings. It's just that I don't have a whole lot of either anymore. I can finish in just a few minutes," said Mr. P., as he laughed.

Her Dad's big 3.

Mrs. S. is 58 years old.

She has three siblings.

All graduated from college and 3 of the 4 have a master's or higher degree as well.

They were the first in their entire family tree to have gone to college.

Their dad always told them three things:

Go to school, get an education, and don't ever let anyone to make you feel like a fool.

Her two sons went to college as well and have been gainfully employed since graduating.

Her dad started a great tradition.

Pumped up.

Mr. M. is an amazingly resilient person.

He's been quadriplegic since 1990 after diving into a lake headfirst, to cool off, after a long hot day at work.

He's used a condom style urinary catheter for many years.

He had a penile implant placed years ago to increase the girth of his penis to enable the condom catheter to stay in place easier.

I had never come across this before, but it made perfect sense.

He laughed when noting the implant has never been used for the intended purpose.

He laughed again when he noted his penis looks more impressive than it would look without the implant in place.

5th time the charm.

Mr. and Mrs. P. have been married for 35 years. He's 68 years old and she's 56. It was his 5th marriage and her 3rd.

I did some quick math: he was 33 years old when he got married for the fifth time and she was 21 when she got married for the third time.

He said he loved to travel to California to pan for gold every year.

I think he was just trying to cut down on the expense of all the engagement and wedding rings!

True or untrue?

The National Care Planning Council has a website with some thought-provoking sections.

The American Perspective on Aging and Health and Americans' Attitudes on Aging is one such section:

"American society in general glorifies youth and fears or even despises old age. This is not the case in many other societies where age is associated with wisdom, knowledge, and special status. In films and on TV old people are often depicted as weak, indecisive, bumbling or even comic. It is rarely that we see older people depicted as decisive, strong, or as leaders. Retirement is presumably a reward for many years of dedication and hard work, but the underlying philosophy is more likely based on the idea that older workers are no longer productive or useful. Instead of taking the role as leaders in their families or in the community as is the case in some countries, the elderly in our country, even after successful careers in earlier years, simply become invisible. They waste their prodigious talents traveling, entertaining, socializing, watching TV or playing golf."

I'm conflicted. I look forward to traveling, socializing, and playing golf but I also don't want to waste my prodigious talents!

Full disclosure: I did need to briefly re-review the definition of prodigious!

His second choice in 1943.

Mr. H. is an 88-year-old WWII veteran.

He had a long career in the Army.

Me: How did you decide on the Army?

Mr. H.: When I enlisted, I was asked if I wanted to be in the Army or the Navy. I said the Navy. The officer responded, "Okay, the Army it is." I wasn't feeling confident enough to speak up at the time but like the rest of my life, God has always shown me the way.

Young at heart.

Mr. C. is 92 years old.

He lives on the 6th floor of a senior living complex.

He seems like an amazingly sociable man but reports spending most of the time alone in his apartment.

The facility has a lot of activities planned but he rarely takes part.

"Everyone is just so old," he says.

I jokingly remind him of his own age.

He clarifies, "Everyone acts and thinks so old. Age is just a number. I'm just tired of people spending all their time talking about how bad things are compared to how they used to be and about all their ailments and upcoming doctor's appointments. It's depressing."

My mother thinks the same way. It's why she says she will never consider moving to a retirement community.

If there was a senior complex that had rules concerning not "acting old," both Mr. C. and my mother might be much happier.

Rich memories.

Mr. C. was a very successful businessperson for many years.

He owned a restaurant/night club in Torrance, California for 27 years as well as a bowling alley/lounge, a jewelry store, and a women's ready to wear clothing store.

He never smoked or drank alcohol and kept himself in good shape over the years by playing racquetball three days a week, boxing, and swimming.

He had one vice, however, gambling.

He lost almost everything gambling on sports.

He's now 92 years old and lives in a 400 square foot studio apartment.

Almost all the wall space is taken up with photo collages that his daughter put together. There are pictures of him with all the famous people who frequented his establishments over the years: Frank Sinatra, Sammy Davis, Dean Martin, Sonny Liston, the Ink Spots, members of the Los Angeles Rams, etc.

He's one of the richest persons I've ever meet in terms of wonderful memories.

He gets a glint in his eye when reminiscing.

He's thankful for having had such a great life.

All smiles.

Mr. S. is 92 years old and very dependent on his wife of over 40 years for his care.

It was a second marriage for both.

She's about thirty years younger.

I commented that she's doing an amazing job of caring for him.

She responded, "He was in his 50s and I was in my 20s when we met. I had a three-year-old boy and a good for nothing husband who was a womanizer. I prayed to God and said if you can help me find a man to love me and help raise my boy, I will be a great wife. He's a beautiful man and he gave us a beautiful life. I'm so thankful. I will do anything for him. All I can do is give him my enduring thanks and loyalty."

Mr. S. grinned and whispered something. I asked him to repeat what he had said. "My first wife never smiled, so the first time I saw her big smile I knew I wanted her in my life."

He smiled. She smiled also.

Not so small anymore.

89-year-old Mrs. L. looks so small, sitting in her recliner, at the assisted living facility where she lives. Hanging on the wall, over the chair, is a picture of her in a military uniform during WWII.

"What branch of the military were you in?" I inquired.

"The Marines," she replied.

"What years active duty?"

"1943 to 1946. I started at Hunter College in NY and then went to Camp Lejeune and worked as a clerk."

Honestly, I didn't know woman were in the Marines during WWII. She didn't look so small anymore!

Military history web sites report The Marine Corps Women's Reserve Schools opened in July 1943. Officer candidates and recruits in training at Mount Holyoke and Hunter Colleges were transferred to Camp Lejeune, where nearly 19,000 women (17,640 enlisted and 820 officers) became Marines during WWII. They were initially taught by reluctant male drill instructors and often subjected to ridicule. However, the woman filled many very important noncombat roles--clerical, parachute riggers, mechanics, radio operators, welders and more.

Drinks not included.

For many years, during the 1950s and 60s, Mr. C. ran a special.

He owned a restaurant/lounge in California.

A $5 ticket would get you a bus ride to and from a Los Angeles Rams home football game, a ticket to the game, and a spaghetti dinner back at his restaurant after the game.

"How were you able to offer such a good price for so many years?"

"I didn't make any money on selling the ticket. The tickets for the game cost me $3 apiece. But folks were happy they were getting such a good deal. I sold liquor to and from the game and back at my place. I made out pretty darn well. I always made some good bucks. Every year I needed to buy more tickets. By the end I was taking over 100 people to every game. It took a long time for others to finally figure out what I was doing. I had a lot of loyal customers. I treated them right and they treated me right. It's really just that simple."

He was just waiting for the right question.

Mr. R. is 87 years-old and doesn't say a whole lot these days.

When I arrived at his home his daughter let me know the same.

He pretty much answered every question I asked with a one- or two-word answer.

"You look like you've been a hard-working man your whole life," I said.

"Been working since I was about 8 years-old," he answered.

A nine-word answer, I thought, let me stay on this line of questioning.

"What kind of work did you do back then?"

"After my parents died, my brother and I were raised by our aunt and uncle in South Carolina. It was a sawmill town. We had a still out back and my brother and I would sell the moonshine through our kitchen window to the men going to and from the sawmill. A 10-cent bumper was a 1/2 pint. A 20-cent bumper was a full pint. I was so small at the time I could barely lift the gallon jug so I would use a funnel and the edge of the table to act as a lever..."

I didn't need to ask any more questions for a while.

It was great to witness.

He seemed so much younger than when I had arrived!

Lucky #9.

Mr. R. is now blind due to end stage glaucoma.

He's hoping he can still find a way to get to and from church.

He's a Pentecostal.

He let me know that his gift is the interpretation of tongues.

I always wondered how that worked.

He filled me in.

He works in tandem with those who possess the gift of "diverse kinds of tongues."

Without tongues there's no need for interpretation.

His gift gives him the ability to interpret tongues.

It's the spirit who gives interpretation of the tongues.

The nine divine gifts of Pentecostalism are: 1. the word of wisdom 2. the word of knowledge 3. faith 4. gifts of healing 5. the working of miracles 6. prophecy 7. discerning of spirits 8. diverse kinds of tongues and 9. the interpretation of tongue.

I plan to have our social worker assist in helping to identify transportation possibilities if his church can't help.

I also hope he's good friends with anyone who possesses gift #4 &/or #5.

His last toenail trimming?

"Is it alright if I trim your toenails?" I asked Mr. R.

He had onychomycosis and onychogryphosis (significantly thickened and deformed toenails) and was complaining about pain in his feet when walking.

"Why would you want to do that?" he asked, "I don't have much longer to live."

His comment, obviously, took me by surprise.

Luckily, as soon as I was about to speak, he let me off the hook.

"Got you tongue tied there for a second or two, didn't I Doc?"

He laughed.

I did too.

White bread.

I've lived in the same town for many years and know a lot of physicians who practice in the area.

A new patient, a 92-year-old man, had previously seen one such acquaintance.

I had obtained some old medical records and remarked to the patient, "I see you've seen Dr.---- previously."

The patient smirked.

"Why are you smiling?" I asked.

"No reason except he's what I would describe as a slice of white bread."

"A slice of white bread? What do you mean?"

"You know, just a plain slice of white bread...no ham and cheese, no peanut butter and jelly...just plain...dull, you know?"

I smiled and let him know I appreciated his honesty and asked for him to let me know if he ever came up with a nickname for me. He laughed.

After he left, I chuckled. His description of the other doctor was right on the money...or the slice.

300 pounds ago...

Mr. M. is 60 years old.

He played baseball in college, was a medic in the military, once fought Chuck Norris in a martial arts contest, and went on to become a nurse while also earning his master's and PhD in Written Communication.

He has written several children's books.

I saw tears welling up in his eyes.

"Are you alright?" I asked, "You've done some great things in your life."

"You're the first doctor, in about twenty years, who has asked me about what I did when I was younger, and thinner. People, even health care professionals, look at me and assume I've always been this way. I haven't always been this weight."

He now weighs over 500 pounds.

He understands that it's a crucial time to get his life back.

I'm hoping the few minutes we spent reviewing his life when he was thinner will allow us to continue to work as a team toward that goal.

Wanted: a good guy.

Roberta is now a companion with Mr. M.

She answered a Craig's list personal ad he had placed a little over two years ago.

She's 62 and Mr. M. is 60.

Mr. M. is functionally impaired from a massive stroke and Roberta does a great job meeting his needs.

She reports that when Mr. M.'s father recently visited he pulled her aside and commented that his son sure is the one benefiting the most from their relationship.

(He was trying to acknowledge all the things she was doing for his son on a day-to-day basis.)

She let him know that she thought it was a 50-50 relationship.

She reported that no man had ever been so kind to her (she had ended a 25-year abusive marriage prior to meeting Mr. M.).

"He's just a good guy. If I had placed an ad, that's what I would have asked for...a good guy."

Much more than just a patient.

Don died last week.

He was 79 years old when he died and led an amazing life.

He was successful in every aspect of his life--as a husband, a father, a decorated college athlete, and as a businessperson.

He was a patient of mine for many years.

Even more, he was a friend.

He also always made it a point to ask about my family when he came in for visits.

He was always a bright spot in an otherwise hectic day in the office.

I was fortunate to have known him for so many years.

Wrong time of the day?

I made a home visit today to see a patient who lives at a nudist colony.

Other residents were out walking, gardening, swimming, bicycle riding, playing tennis, socializing, etc. in the nude.

The effects of age and gravity on the male and female body were very visible.

I was there in the early afternoon, and it was a bright sunny day.

I often joke that I still look okay, by candlelight, when nude.

The same might possibly be true for some of the folks I saw there as well.

Grandpa, it's me, stop doing that.

There's no easy answer to the question:

What can be done about the elderly demented folks who like to wander, escape or who have severe behavioral symptoms associated with dementia (aggressiveness, episodes of anger, psychosis, hallucinations, inappropriateness--walking around nude, urinating or defecating in public, masturbating in front of others, etc.)?

Family members can take turns watching 24/7 but most scattered families don't have the ability to do this.

Families can hire 24/7 care (basically sitters) at a cost of anywhere from $10/hour (for those hired privately) to over $20/hour (for those hired through a licensed, bonded company) for a total cost of approximately $7000-$14,000/month or they can place their loved one in an assisted living facility (that accepts patients with dementia) or a nursing home.

The use of physical restraints (posey vests, etc.) by facilities is no longer acceptable, and if used will generate an ACHA evaluation. The use of medications to attempt to treat (sedative medications, anti-anxiety medications, anti-psychotic medications) is associated with adverse events (falls, hypotension, increased mortality, decreased cognition) and if/when used by facilities will often lead to the appearance of a malpractice attorney representing the family of the patient if there's an adverse event.

It's all actually quite depressing.

Dementia runs in my family. I'm hoping that if/when I become demented, I will keep my social graces and behave so I can stay at home and not be a burden to my family.

In the old days, elderly family members were taken care of by the daughter or the daughter-in-law.

With more women working outside of the home, and smaller families in general, this often is no longer an option for most.

I do think we need to get back to multiple generations living in the same home again. I know this goes against the American dream of leaving home and starting your own life, but no one can usually re-orient a demented older person acting out better than a family member.

That's all he had to say about that.

I asked 92-year-old Mr. H. if he had any hobbies.

He said, "What exactly do you mean?"

I said, "You know, are there any things that you enjoy doing or that bring you joy?"

He said, "I like staying alive. I like to go outside occasionally and sit on the swing. If I get thirsty, I like to drink some water."

He smiled.

I smiled.

I decided to move onto a new topic.

I didn't ask if he was related to Forrest Gump.

It's a great idea (Author unknown)!

Someone shared this with me.

The last wishes of Alexander the Great:

On his death bed, Alexander summoned his generals and told them his three ultimate wishes:

-The best doctors should carry his coffin.

-The wealth he had accumulated (money, gold, precious stones) should be scattered along the procession to the cemetery.

-His hands should be let loose, hanging outside the coffin for all to see.

One of his generals, who was surprised by these unusual requests, asked Alexander to explain.

Here's what Alexander the Great had to say:

I want the best doctors to carry my coffin to demonstrate that, in the face of death, even the best doctors in the world have no power to heal.

I want the road to be covered with my treasure so that everybody sees that material wealth acquired on earth, stays on earth.

I want my hands to swing in the wind, so that people understand that we come to this world empty handed and we leave this world empty handed after the most precious treasure of all is exhausted, and that is TIME.

We do not take to our grave any material wealth, although our good deeds can be our travelers' checks. TIME is our most precious treasure because it is LIMITED. We can produce more wealth, but we cannot produce more time.

When we give someone our time, we give a portion of our life that we will never take back. Our time is our life!

The best present that you can give to your family and friends is your TIME. May God grant you plenty of TIME and may you have the wisdom to give it away so that you can LIVE, LOVE and DIE in peace.

Foreplay.

Mrs. K. has a valid complaint.

She's the wife and primary caregiver for Mr. K.

"I take care of him all day long. He keeps me up most nights hollering out in his sleep and getting up to pace around the house. He wants to try and have sex almost every night, but I have no interest in being intimate with him."

Years ago, I read an article by a sex therapist.

The author noted:

-For many men, foreplay consists of walking across the threshold to the bedroom.

-For many women, foreplay consists of everything that has happened in the previous 24 hours.

This is a perfect example.

Things aren't looking too promising for Mr. K.

The status-quo.

While reviewing some old records, on a 78-year-old patient, I came across an assessment by his previous physician:

"Overall, the patient is status-quo in a state of chronic, semi-well compensated, moderate to severe ill health."

I'll need some time to figure out exactly what it means.

The computer sees nothing!

Mr. C. is 86 years-old and had a stroke years ago that left him completely paralyzed on his left side--his left arm and leg are atrophied and contracted.

I received a follow-up note from a cardiologist who had seen him recently.

Under the general physical exam section, it noted that "no sensory abnormalities were noted, and no motor dysfunction was seen."

There are only two possible explanations:

-The cardiologist examined Mr. C. with his eyes closed.

-The computer-generated template was not amended with the correct information.

Since this seems to happen so often these days, I suspect that #2 it is!

The note was signed at about 11 PM, most certainly after a long day for the cardiologist...just what most litigation attorneys hope for...mistakes.

The Necco king!

Mr. W. is now 93 years old.

He's from Massachusetts and has been a lifelong Necco wafer lover. He can't remember when he hasn't eaten close to a roll a day.

Necco stands for New England Confectionary Company and the wafers, their core product, were first produced in 1847.

During the Civil War they were carried by Union soldiers and were referred to as *hub wafers.*

They were renamed Necco wafers in 1912.

Each roll of Necco wafers contains eight flavors: lemon (yellow), lime (green), orange (orange), clove (purple), cinnamon (white), wintergreen (pink), licorice (black) and chocolate (brown).

My favorite has always been the black.

Mr. W. doesn't have a favorite.

His daughter has a lot on her plate as his caregiver but luckily has found a local store that makes sure to keep the Neccos in stock now that Mr. W. lives with her in Florida.

He currently has a plastic bag with rolls on his bedside table.

It looked like at least a two-week supply.

Italia!

Mr. C. wanted to let me know that there are only two types of people in the world.

"Those who are Italian and those who want to be Italian."

"Why?" I asked.

"Because we have the best skin, the best-looking woman, the best food, and the best music."

He's 83 years old and has advanced dementia.

I nodded to show I agreed and let him know I love Italian food.

He smiled.

Things really weren't that great prior to the fall.

Mr. B. is 93 years old.

Two years ago (at age 91) he fell out of a bed, during a stay at a rehab facility, after his third major cardiac surgery. He broke a hip and continues to walk slowly and only with the assist of a walker.

Litigation against the facility is ongoing. A settlement has been offered, but not accepted by the family's lawyer.

Over the years, prior to this most recent surgery and fall, he had suffered two heart attacks, three strokes, had a partial colectomy for colon cancer, had been treated for prostate cancer and had major orthopedic intervention after two serious car accidents.

He was already significantly functionally impaired but his wife feels the fall was a result of negligence on the part of the facility and that "his life has been ruined" because of the fall.

I decided to not review his significant past medical history and poor functionality prior to the fall at the rehab facility.

It most likely would not alter her thoughts or the desire of the family lawyer to continue litigating for the greatest monetary settlement possible.

Painful steps.

Mr. M. is 60 years-old, 5'9" and weighs 493 pounds.

His BMI is 72.8.

He needs to have an elective surgery performed.

He was told by the plastic surgeon that he requires a BMI of 38 or below before he will be a candidate for the surgery.

He will need to get down to 258 pounds or less-he needs to lose 52.3% of his current body weight.

I'm not sure he really has any idea just how difficult a task this will be to accomplish.

I decided that now was not the time to remind him of that fact.

He just needs to take it one step at a time--even though each step is painful due to his severe knee and hip arthritis.

Three out of four brothers.

Mr. A. was medically discharged after his 5th tour in Vietnam with multiple shrapnel injuries. He was awarded multiple Purple Hearts, Bronze, and Silver stars and a Distinguished Service Cross during his service.

Mr. A.'s older brother was killed while serving in Vietnam.

One of Mr. A.'s younger brothers lost a leg after stepping on a land mine in Vietnam.

All were in the Army.

"How old are you?" he asked me.

"53," I replied.

"I'm glad you were too young to go to Vietnam," he said, "You're the same age as my youngest brother. He never had to go either."

"Thanks to you and your family for your service and sacrifices."

Lifesaver.

Mr. Z. is 90 years old and has some cognitive impairment.

He has complete recall, however, concerning July 25, 1956.

He was a 33-year-old radio operator on a cargo vessel that was carrying a load of bananas back to New York City from Costa Rica.

He was the first to hear the S.O.S. from the SS Andrea Doria after it collided with the Swedish ocean liner, the Stockholm, off the coast of Nantucket.

Over 50 people died but his actions were instrumental in alerting others to allow the rescue efforts to get underway as quickly as possible.

He acknowledges that day as being one of the most significant days of his life.

I completely agreed.

Loving green.

Mr. Z. spent over 20 years working on a cargo ship making the trip from New York to Central America and back for the Chiquita Banana company during the mid-1950's to the late 1970's.

Each round trip would take two to three weeks. He would be home for a week and then head back out. He never missed a trip due to illness and never took an extended vacation.

It brought up the obvious question.

"Do you like bananas?"

"I can't stand bananas. I can't even stand to look at them. The only good thing about bananas is that they allowed me to earn a good living for many years. They were green when we picked them up--the same color as money."

He laughed and so did I.

Back in the day, I'm sure he laughed all the way to the bank.

One of the greatest.

Maximino is an 82-year-old man.

I mentioned he was the first Maximino I had ever met.

He let me know it's not a common first name for a reason. It originated as an Italian name and means the "greatest."

"There can't be too many of the greatest walking around you know (he smiled, and I agreed)!"

I believe.

I went to a conference recently.

One of the talks was on the high percentage of marijuana and heroin use by members of the armed forces while serving in Vietnam.

I saw a Vietnam veteran today.

Amid taking his history I asked him about the drug culture during his time in Southeast Asia.

He remembers what he was told by a member of his unit when he first arrived in Vietnam:

"Man made booze, God made grass; I believe in God. Do you believe in God?"

He went on to say, "I was 18, scared to death, and looked up to those guys. I started smoking marijuana soon after I arrived."

One of the amazing WAVES.

Mrs. V. was part of the WAVES--Women Accepted for Voluntary Emergency Services-in WWII.

The official name was the U.S. Naval Women's Reserve, but the nickname stuck.

She was 25 years old at the time and, due to her previous education and training as a schoolteacher, was put in charge of running the women's living quarters while stationed at the Naval Training School in Georgia.

She served for 2 and 1/2 years.

She's now 96 years old and crippled with arthritis but is still very quick witted.

Once she got rolling, it was one funny or sarcastic comment after another.

I was cracking up and she had a satisfied smirk on her face.

The presence of women in the military was very controversial in the 1940s and many, even though they were performing vital duties at home to free up men to fight overseas, were subjected to ridicule and crude remarks.

I suspect her wit and sarcasm served her well back then and that many men left an encounter with her with the short end of the stick.

Music for romance.

Mr. C. has been sick for a while.

He lost a lot of weight, but his wife reported she knows he's starting to improve.

"How do you know?" I asked.

"Two reasons," she stated, "he recently started to play his guitar again, which he hadn't wanted to do the entire time he was ill, and his penis is starting to grow and get hard again. It was shriveling up while he was ill. We're both glad to see it starting to come around again," she said with a grin.

He's 82 years old and they've been married almost 60 years.

I think her clues to his recovery are probably as good as, or much better than, any sophisticated medical test could possibly be.

All 3-in-1 day.

Mr. and Mrs. S. have been married for 61 years.

Although Mrs. S. was not Catholic (Mr. S. was), they went to a Catholic church as a family, throughout their marriage and their children were brought up in the Catholic church.

She never took part in the Sacrament of the Eucharist--Communion.

When she was in her 70's she decided to join. She reports being Baptized and going through First Holy Communion and Confirmation all on the same day.

"It was a busy day," and she reports to being a little embarrassed, "with everyone watching," since it was Easter Sunday.

She laughs when she says she suspects the priest wanted to make sure she didn't change her mind.

Their song.

Nearing the end of my visit I had concluded that 83-year-old Mr. E. and 75-year-old Mrs. E. had a very poor quality of life.

I didn't verbalize my thoughts.

He's been bed-bound and poorly responsive for a couple of years, after a series of devastating strokes, and she's been his 24/7 devoted caregiver.

He spends his days in a hospital bed.

She sleeps in a single bed in the same room in case he needs anything during the night.

Their bedroom was filled with his medications, creams, incontinence garments, and pads.

"Can I show you something?" she asked.

"Of course."

She gently shook her husband's shoulders until he opened his eyes. "Honey, honey, I love you..."

"A bushel and a peck and a hug around the neck," said Mr. E., as clear as day.

"Why are you the luckiest man in the world?" she then asked him.

"Because I'm married to you," he said with a slight grin.

Mrs. E. smiled as she stroked his hair while he closed his eyes and drifted back off to sleep.

"That was really great, thank you."

"Oh, it's just something we've done since we were married," she said.

They recently celebrated their 55th wedding anniversary.

It was also another excellent reminder to not be so quick to judge a person's quality of life.

I wasn't expecting this response.

Mr. and Mrs. M. are proud of being "simple country folk."

They have thick southern accents.

They both talk really, really s----l----o----w.

I asked them about their children.

Mrs. M. answered.

"My oldest son lives up in Pennsylvania with his family...he's a nuclear engineer. My oldest daughter lives a few miles from here with her family... she's a family nurse practitioner. My youngest lives in the next town over with her family...she's the chief of pharmacy at the regional hospital."

To be completely honest, I wasn't expecting an answer such as this.

It was awesome!

A room with family?

Mr. W. is an 85-year-old man who lives in an assisted living facility.

He has severe dementia, but it hasn't stopped him from socializing.

His social graces are intact, and he gets a sparkle in his eyes when being engaged in conversation.

He responds to all questions with an answer that has nothing to do with the question that was asked.

"How are you doing today?" I ask.

"You bet I do. Back when I owned a bar in Hartford Connecticut I pretty much did everything so that's why I have twenty-one shirts now, all different colors, for when I worked for the post office, and I only get one egg and a piece of toast for my music."

"Are you happy with the food here?" I then ask.

"Not as well as I used to 'cause I've got one bad ear and I like to walk as much as I can, and I had a good bowel movement today and I wish we had a better television in our room."

This went on for a while.

His vital signs and general physical exam were all stable.

"You have a great day," I say while shaking his hand preparing to leave.

"Are you going to take me with you?" he inquires.

"You have a great day also."

My response obviously didn't answer his question either.

He had a big smile on his face when I left.

I was sort of bummed on my way back to the office again trying to contemplate why he doesn't have a family member, somewhere, who would open their home to him.

I think of this frequently whenever I leave an ALF.

Good for business?

The pharmacy near our home now has a small health clinic.

The sign out front of the store advises folks driving by to "come on in to get healthy at our health clinic."

The sign also had the following specials noted underneath the message to get healthy:

Ice Cream 2/$6.00

Lays Chips 2/$3.00
Coke 2/$2.50

I couldn't help but smile.

Hard knocks.

I had the pleasure of meeting Joe yesterday.

Joe is a former NFL running back.

We briefly talked about the recent NFL settlement for 765 million dollars for the former players and families regarding information that was reportedly hidden pertaining to the potential long-term effects of head trauma and multiple concussions.

Joe played for a total of 5 years and is getting a small NFL pension.

He's now 71 years old.

He has some evident word finding difficulties and he had me introduce myself three times to help him remember my name.

I did not ask him the one question I would have loved to ask:

"If you had known about the potential effects of head trauma and concussions, would you have still played nonetheless?"

I'm sure he would have said yes.

A cure for what ails ya!

Mr. M. is my age.

He's been quadriplegic since an accident in 1990.

He was back home after another hospitalization and a close call with death.

He was septic but responded to fluid resuscitation and intravenous antibiotics.

He's back to his baseline.

He still has a glint in his eye, loves to joke and make sarcastic comments, and is so looking forward to his favorite outing in the whole world...traveling in his electric wheelchair to get donuts about 1/4 mile from his home.

He's got a better outlook on life than most neurologically intact folks I know.

I'd been feeling sorry for myself lately due to a post-cold hacking cough for a couple of weeks.

I didn't feel that way after my visit with Mr. M.

Not so little anymore.

Mr. D. was married to Big Red for over 50 years.

(Photos confirmed that his wife had a full head of red hair!)

They had 7 children together.

She spent years caring for him after a devastating stroke.

She unexpectedly died before he did.

Their youngest daughter, nick-named Little Red, is now his caregiver.

(She also has a red hair!)

She also takes care of her older disabled brother (after an injury), her two high-need stepchildren (both with fetal alcohol syndrome), and her disabled 27-year-old son (after a severe MVA at age 16).

Her husband helps whenever he can but is out working multiple jobs to provide.

She admits to some tough times emotionally but, in general, appears filled with an incredible sense of gratitude.

Big Red would be very proud of Little Red!

Staying put.

Mr. M. is 97 years-old, and Mrs. M. is 96.

They still live, for the most part, independently in a townhouse with assistance, for only 3 hours a day, from a home health agency.

They have been married for 77 years.

They did not have children.

Before I could ask, they commented that many health care professionals over the years have recommended they move to an assisted living facility.

I decided to not join the ranks of the many.

On my drive back to the office I had two thoughts:

    1. 77 years!

2.   What an amazing couple!

Hiding amongst a bunch of other questions.

Included in a 70-year-old's medical records was his military discharge medical exam performed in 1965.

Prior to the physical exam were a series of 50 questions:

While active duty did you suffer from any of the following?

1.   Joint pain?
2.   Trouble breathing?
3.   Neuritis?
4.   Homosexual tendencies?
5.   Visual problems?
6.   Hearing related concerns?
7.   → 50. etc.

I suspect the answer to #4, in 1965, was always "No."

The discharge form used these days does not have question #4.

Home sweet home.

Mr. H. had a devastating stroke in April.

He's 82 years-old, unable to talk, swallow effectively, or move one side of his body.

He's at home surrounded by family pictures and his pet birds.

One of his four children is always there to assist his 80-year-old wife with his care.

The children are taking turns flying in from other parts of the country and stay two-four weeks at a time.

There are no plans for Mr. H. to go to a nursing home.

"Where we are from (a Caribbean Island)," says his daughter, "there is no such thing as a nursing home. We take care of our own."

She said this as she was helping to re-position her father in his bed after assisting her mom in giving him a bed bath.

I'm certain there are a lot of folks in nursing homes who wish they would have been born in the Caribbean and into this family.

Knowing they are loved.

A good friend recently commented that he has always felt guilty about placing his mother in a nursing home prior to her death.

I completely understand how he's feeling.

Every situation is different.

Not all families can keep a loved one at home.

Sleep deprivation and other issues (behavioral issues of dementia--outbursts, impulsivity, loss of social graces, sun-downing, absence of multiple caregivers, incontinence, etc.) can completely wear down the most motivated of caregivers and render attempts at home care problematic and dangerous.

Given a multitude of factors, including the ones mentioned above, keeping his mom at home near the end of her life was not possible for him.

I'm sure my friends mother knew how much she was loved.

This is the most important thing at the end of life.

A peckerologist.

A 70-year-old male wanted to know if he should go see a "penis-machinist."

He laughed.

I did also.

I then asked how he had come up with that name for a urologist.

"My wife used to get annoyed whenever I would call him a peckerologist, so I needed to come up with another name."

An uplifting tale (forwarded by my brother)-Author unknown.

A 92-year-old, well-poised and proud man, who is fully dressed each morning by eight o'clock, with his hair fashionably combed and shaved perfectly, even though he is legally blind, moved to a nursing home today.

His wife of 70 years recently passed away, making the move necessary. After many hours of waiting patiently in the lobby of the nursing home, he smiled sweetly when told his room was ready.

As he maneuvered his walker to the elevator, I provided a visual description of his tiny room.

"I love it," he stated with the enthusiasm of an eight-year-old having just been presented with a new puppy.

"Mr. Jones, you haven't seen the room; just wait..."

"That doesn't have anything to do with it," he replied.

"Happiness is something you decide on ahead of time.

Whether I like my room or not doesn't depend on how the furniture is arranged...it's how I arrange my mind. I already decided to love it.

It's a decision I make every morning when I wake up. I have a choice; I can spend the day in bed recounting the difficulty I have with the parts of my body that no longer work or get out of bed and be thankful for the ones that do.

Each day is a gift, and if my eyes open, I'll focus on the new day and all the happy memories I've stored away...just for this time in my life...

Old age is like a bank account. You withdraw from what you've put in.

So, my advice to you would be to deposit a lot of happiness in the bank account of memories!

I'm still depositing."

"Remember the five simple rules to be happy:

1.   Free your heart from hatred.

2. Free your mind from worries.

3. Live simply.

4. Give more.

5. Expect less."

Medications to the rescue!

Mr. B. is a 76-year-old with a steady girlfriend for the last 6 months.

"She's a much younger woman—she's 66."

He inquired about what options might be available to allow him to perform intimately again.

I first inquired if they had decided on this together.

"She's ready," he said, "she just told to make sure I got something that would at least let me finish whatever I started."

A memorable face.

On meeting 85 y/o Mr. W. for the first time I said, "It's great to put a face to your name."

I have no idea why I chose this as an opening line.

About 15 minutes later, while still taking his medical history, he said, "I gotta ask ya quickly, did my face disappoint you?"

He laughed.

"I'm sorry, why would you ask that," I replied.

He then reminded me of my opening comment.

We both laughed and I quickly determined I didn't need to ask him any short-term recall questions to test his memory.

I left the encounter grinning at the fact that the same couldn't be said for me.

Still brings grins.

Mr. F. let me know he tricked his wife into thinking he was wealthy before they married because he dressed well and had a nice car.

His wife grinned.

He reports that it wasn't until later that she found out his nickname for most of his life had been "All Show, No Dough."

They are now in their 90s.

I'm sure he has told this story numerous times over their 65 years of marriage but seeing them both laugh, after all these years, was still awesome.

One-armed bandits.

I hadn't seen Mr. A. for a while, and he just sort of seemed out of it.

He was still in bed when I got to his house at about 10 AM.

He's 78 years old and previously had a major stroke, but I was worried he had something acute taking place that was making him so drowsy.

After examining him I relayed my concerns to his wife who had been standing next to me the whole time.

"I'm a little worried about your husband. I'm thinking I might need to run a few tests to try and see if everything is all right," I said to Mrs. A.

"Oh, he's okay," said Mrs. A., "he just had an exciting night. We didn't get back from the Hard Rock Casino until a few hours ago. He's just still sleepy. He didn't get to bed until after 4 AM."

She let me know that he could still play the slot machines without any trouble (his previous stroke had "only" left him paralyzed on one side of his body).

I wasn't expecting her comment.

I had noticed a new handicapped accessible minivan in their driveway but hadn't mentioned it and Mrs. A. decided not to mention being out till the early morning "partying" when I arrived.

I was smiling most of the drive back to the office thinking about them at the casino.

The balls are still in play.

Three dads (including me) were talking at a Christmas party gathering at my daughter's riding barn.

One of the dad's had two young children running around.

Another asked him if he was going to have more kids.

"No," he replied, "I'm a gelding. I used to be a stallion but now I'm a gelding."

We all laughed.

We determined that we were now all geldings.

We shared some more laughs reminiscing about our vasectomies; we even hammed it up whenever our wives came by.

On the way home I got a reality check from my wife.

"At least you only had your tubes cut. Stallions have their balls cut off," she reminded me.

"Yep, you're right about that!"

Sicker than I thought?

"I'm going to need to have some labs drawn, when possible," I mentioned to the nurse as I was about to leave the patient's home.

"Are you a heart stick?" I heard the nurse, who was originally from the Caribbean (and still had a strong accent), ask the patient.

I stopped at the door.

"What? I don't understand," said the patient.

"Has anyone ever told you that you were a heart stick?" the nurse repeated.

"I don't think I've ever had a heart stick," said the patient.

I walked back into the room. "She wants to know if you are a hard stick, h-a-r-d. If it's ever been hard to draw your blood in the past."

"Oh...I don't think so. Thanks for clarifying."

Happy tears.

Mr. G. is 87 years old and has advanced dementia.

I saw him recently for a medical evaluation.

His wife is his devoted caregiver and showed me many pictures of their children and extended families.

They have a beautiful family.

Mrs. G. wanted me to know more about this man who now has a great difficulty in communicating.

"I married my first husband at age 16 and we had 4 children. He died unexpectedly from a brain hemorrhage. I didn't know what I would do. Rob was a college professor. We fell in love and got married two years later. The kids were all still so young. We've been married for 54 years, and he's been a wonderful father. We had a family celebration at our 40th wedding anniversary and everyone wanted us to give a speech. Rob's was short. He wanted to thank two people: my mother for giving birth to me and my first husband for being the biological father of his 4 amazing children. There was not a dry eye in the room that day."

There was still not a dry eye in the room.

Microwave Joe.

When asked if he's still preparing his own meals, 91-year-old Joe C. reports that his nickname for many decades has been Microwave Joe.

His daughter either makes meals for him that he can reheat in the microwave, or she purchases ready-made meals for which he can do the same.

He thinks he might have had one of the original microwave ovens.

He remembers it being called the "Radarange."

Some quick research shows that, in 1967, Raytheon offered for sale the first popular in-home countertop microwave oven: the "Radarange."

It sold then for almost $500, close to roughly $4500 in today's dollars.

So, it's easy to make a couple of conclusions:

1. Since about age 49 he's been microwave Joe.
2. Back then he was rolling in the dough!

He paid it forward.

Mr. and Mrs. W. adopted a boy who was 2 years old and significantly disabled due to cerebral palsy. His son is now 30 and working full time as an executive chef after graduating from high school, college, and culinary school.

Mr. and Mrs. W. adopted a girl who was abandoned at age 3 by her drug dependent/abusing parents. She is now thirty-five and has a family of her own.

Mr. W. is now eighty-seven and totally dependent, for the last 5 years, due to an unfortunate series of health-related events.

His son and daughter go to great lengths to help Mrs. W. care for Mr. W.

Both have nothing but wonderful things to say about their father and how he went to such great lengths to provide for them despite their less-than-optimal starts in life.

They let me know they will go to great lengths to help provide for him in his time of need and to make this stage of his life as wonderful as possible.

Mr. W. doesn't say much these days, but I'm sure I saw him smile when he overheard this discussion.

Anniversary bling times two.

Mr. and Mrs. G have been married 63 years. They let me know they have had 126 wedding anniversaries.

"Why? " I asked.

"We got married while I was stationed in Japan on December 28th at the American consulate, but it wasn't recorded by the Bureau of Statistics until January 5th because the offices were closed for the holidays."

"It's been nice. We've celebrated twice each year, with a cake and a gift, to mark the anniversary of both dates."

Mrs. G. was wearing a lot of jewelry!

Recreating my mouth.

I came across a note by a recreational therapist in a medical record on a patient.

The patient was a 93-year-old man.

"Talking and reminiscing" were noted in the section entitled "Recreational activities performed today."

Starting now I will remind all that I'm not just talking--I'm recreating!

Still valid.

A staff member let me know one of our patients had "expired." I thanked him for letting me know our patient had died.

Memberships and warranties expire (to end or to no longer be valid).

People die (to pass from physical life).

So much more than a snack.

One of my favorite snacks growing-up were Devil Dogs.

I recently met Mr. C., a 77-year-old.

He was a Devil Dog in Vietnam from 1967-1968.

The moniker of Devil Dogs for US Marines was reportedly bestowed upon them by the Germans in 1918, due to the Marines fighting with such tenacity that they were likened to "Dogs from Hell." The Devil Dogs arrived in Vietnam in 1966.

Military sites document that they engaged in some of the bloodiest and most intense fighting.

Mr. C. has dealt with flashbacks and other symptoms of PTSD since them, including an element of guilt due to being one of the few from his Squadron, who made it home.

He still intermittently tears up.

He struggled for years emotionally, had some setbacks in his personal life, but is proud to have great children, to finally be happily married and to have been a very successful businessperson.

Like so many other Veterans, I wish he would record some of the things he experienced as a teenager while serving.

I tried to subtly encourage him to do just that.

Another first.

Recently met a 76-year-old man who lives at a retirement community.

During the review of systems, I asked him if he was sexually active.

"Yes…extremely," he replied.

He went on to explain that he's one of only two single men so there's a significant need for his "services" from many of the widowed or divorced women who reside there.

I wasn't expecting his response and was, frankly, initially sort of stunned.

Surprisingly, he wasn't on any medications for erections.

Laughing, congratulating, or admonishing him didn't seem appropriate—we had just met!

He noted he was always practicing safe sex.

I asked him to review his definition of safe sex.

He said all the right things.

At the end of our visit, I reminded him to continue to be careful.

I may have additional thoughts before our next visit now that I know how frequently his services are required.

Nailed it.

I saw a cartoon of an old man down on one knee, proposing to what looked like a much younger woman.

He had the ring box opened, revealing a huge diamond ring.

The caption read, "Would you be my primary caregiver?"

I couldn't help but laugh.

Interesting advertising.

A six-story senior complex I visited had the following sign out front:

"Life begins here!"

When I got back to the office, I looked up their website to learn more about the facility.

The opening statement on their web page noted "If you lived here, you would be within minutes from the hospital and a wide assortment of medical specialists."

I smiled when I linked this statement to the sign out front of the facility.

Only a nonagenarian.

Mrs. C. is 82 years old, the youngest of 4 children.

She has a brother who is 96, and two sisters who are 86 and 87.

Her mother lived to be 108 years old.

"My dad died young…he was only 93."

She didn't smile or laugh, so neither did I.

Longevity is clearly a serious topic in her family!

Just one will do.

63-year-old Mr. C. is chronically ill with cirrhosis and is on the transplant list for a liver.

He appears significantly older than his chronological age.

He's fallen a couple of times recently.

He declined to accept a cane or walker to increase his base of support.

"Why?" I asked.

"I don't want to look too old."

I couldn't help but smile.

Finally, he grinned as well.

"Don't you think a severe head injury from a fall might make you less likely to receive a transplant?" I asked.

He grinned again.

"What are your thoughts?" I continued.

"I'm just trying to figure out how many canes or walkers I'll need."

"Let's just start with one of each."

Thankfully, he agreed.

I cannot determine the extent of my injuries at this time.

The most common advertisements on billboards these days, in and around Orlando, are from attorneys.

Three signs seen recently:

You fall…you call.

Accidente de auto?

My attorney got me $1 million dollars.

I always do some quick math in my head to determine the attorney's 35 to 40 percent cut of the "got me" dollars.

I wonder why they don't include that amount in big letters on the billboards as well?

He has decided against.

"I discussed the risk of surgery that includes but are not limited to anesthesia complications that may lead to death, cardiopulmonary arrest that may lead to death, and sepsis that again may lead to death. The patient does not want to take the risk. He has decided against being further evaluated for surgery at this time."

After the above consultation with a surgeon, a patient of mine no longer wished to be evaluated for an elective hernia repair.

He had multiple, serious, complex, underlying medical issues.

The hernia was easily reducible and relatively asymptomatic, but he and his family were insistent on being evaluated for an elective repair, despite my advice against the same.

The surgeon's expertly worded discussion helped to bolster my counsel.

The Last Lecture.

Prior to his death at age 47 from pancreatic cancer, Randy Pausch gave *The Last Lecture*. These are some of my favorite quotes of his:

-We cannot change the cards we are dealt, just how we play the hand.

-The key question to keep asking is, are you spending your time on the right things? Because time is all you have.

-Showing gratitude is one of the simplest yet most powerful things humas can do for each other.

-Never, ever underestimate the importance of having fun.

-I am going to keep having fun every day I have left, because there is no other way of life. You just have to decide whether you are a Tigger or an Eeyore.

My path to doctoring

My mom's side of the family was medical. Her dad was a doctor, as are her twin brothers.

My dad's side was not medical. Both he and his dad were engineers.

I wasn't sure what I wanted to major in when I applied to college, even though I enjoyed a biology course I took my senior year of high school, which included doing operations on rats.

My three older siblings were all attending the University of Virginia (UVA).

Since I always did well in math and science and literally sucked at foreign languages, I applied to the engineering school at UVA.

I was accepted.

Soon after school started, I realized I shared classes with some incredibly talented people.

I vividly remember one of my first engineering science labs.

There was a box of wires, switches, transducers, and capacitors on the table, and we were told to build a radio.

While I was still on some of the initial steps many of my classmates were already tuning into stations.

Also, soon after starting college, I began to work part time as a respiratory therapy technician (RT Tech) at the University Hospital.

My parents then moved from Pelham, New York to Charlottesville, Virginia during the spring of my 1st year. Their decision to move allowed me to eventually be reclassified as an in-state student and, even more importantly, enabled me to work full time during school breaks and summers as an RT Tech.

It became apparent to me that my interest and aptitude for the human body was much greater than my interest in many of the engineering concepts I was working hard to understand.

By my second year of college, I decided I wanted to pursue a medical career. I had an excellent faculty advisor who was able to help me map out a way I could graduate in four years with an engineering degree while at the same time completing all the course work needed to be eligible to apply to medical school.

However, I could not take the Medical College Admission Test (MCAT) until December of my fourth year, when I had finished all the prerequisite courses. Most "pre-meds" had taken the MCAT in the spring of their third year.

My medical school application was not considered complete until the scores were available.

In those days, one could reserve a spot in a medical school class with a very nominal fee.

By the time my application was complete, most of the incoming classes were filled. I got rejected by three medical schools and was put on the waiting list at two.

During my time working as an RT Tech, I often worked alongside Cardiovascular Technicians (CV Tech's). Near the end of my 4th year of college I was offered, and accepted, a transfer to be a CV Tech.

I had an excellent job for at least the next year, since it didn't look likely I would get into an entering medical school class.

However, the day before my first final exam, I got a phone call from the UVA Medical School admission dean offering me a spot.

It was the time of year that many who had reserved spots began to release their holds when they finally determined exactly where they wanted to attend.

He also gave me feedback that it was my letters of recommendation from my supervisors at the hospital that had allowed me to leapfrog over many on the waiting list.

Obviously, I accepted the offer.

During undergraduate reunions I have always thanked friends and acquaintances of mine who had gotten into UVA Medical School, for relinquishing their hold to attend another medical school, so I could be offered a spot.

After graduating from medical school in 1985, I did a three-year family medicine residency, then a two-year geriatric fellowship, then spent three years on the faculty of the family medicine residency program, and finally, moved and joined a practice--a multi-specialty group practice--in Florida, for five years.

I then started working for the Department of Veterans Affairs in 1998 and, other than a 3-month absence some years ago, have been there ever since.

"Medicine allows us to participate in the lives of others…It is an advantage and trust given to a few-and none of us can take that for granted. Be humbled by the honor."-George S. Poehlman MD

I remain humbled and thankful for the privilege of being a physician.

Some additional thoughts

I did residency at a time when there were no rules regarding the number of hours in a row a resident could work.

Being on-duty for thirty-six hours or more was the norm for a resident when on-call; a rite of passage in one's journey.

Most clinical rotations were three-month blocks.

Some clinical rotations required in-house call every other night or at most every third night.

In 1989, the Bell Commission Report implicated the long work hours of residents as a contributory cause that led to the death of a patient.

Since 2003 the Accreditation Council for Graduate Medical Education (ACGME) created guidelines for resident work hours "to promote safe care and high-quality learning."

The ACGME now mandates limiting total work hours in a week, ensuring at least one day off a week, only working a maximum of twenty-four hours in a row and in-house call frequency of no more than every three days, averaged over four weeks.

Some feel this has adversely affected the clinical experience and competency acquired during one's residency training and worry it has promoted more of a shift-work mentality in younger physicians.

Nonetheless, the mandates by the ACGME were necessary.

I also trained and initially practiced before the electronic health record (EHR) came into existence. The EHR has many benefits, but it can also have a negative impact on a clinician-patient encounter.

I wrote the following article on this topic in *Physicians Practice* over ten-years ago and still have many of the same thoughts:

Like many other middle-aged physicians, I used to have recurring negative thoughts about my practice's EHR:

-Please make it go away.
-Maybe I'll retire before I really need to start using all aspects of the EHR.

In an article in Family Practice News, the authors (Dr. Skolnik and Dr. Wilkinson) raised three excellent questions regarding the use of the EHR:

1. Will technology interfere with the humanism and patient interactions that form the heart and soul--if not the science--of medical care?

2. Will placement of a screen in the room divert the physician from giving direct attention to the patient in favor of inputting required data?

3. Will the "narrative" of the illness--the description of the patient experience--be lost as the representation of the disease is narrowed to discrete data fields?

The EHR, in some form, is here to stay. However, when it comes to the use of computers, many physician practices clearly lag-behind the rest of the world and our society.

Here are a couple of typical statements I've heard from patients:

"I didn't tell the nurse I was depressed because she never looked at me when she asked the question. I figured she didn't really care."

"I want to see a different specialist. He just kept his head down typing the whole time. He's a computer doctor, not a real doctor."

I've tried hard to not allow the EHR to adversely affect the physician-patient relationship. Here's my approach after settling in with the EHR over the last few years:

1.   Every visit still starts and ends with a personal interaction. It doesn't take long to briefly socialize by asking about a patient's family, occupation, and/or hobby. I also always make sure to include short periods of non-computer use because eye contact with patients and an understanding nod are not part of the EHR.

2.   I evaluated the physical design of my exam rooms. I've seen some offices in which the physical layout of the room is less than optimal, due to the physician having his back to the patient and/or the family members at times. Obviously, a layout such as this does not allow for ideal nonverbal communication.

3.   If I sense tension in the room during a difficult patient encounter, I've found it best to move away from the computer. Unless I move away, the tendency is to keep my head down looking at the monitor for answers that usually aren't going to be found on the computer screen.

4.   I remember that it's an advantage and a disadvantage for patients/families and others to easily read my records, compared to hand-written notes from "the old days." Medico-legally, if it wasn't recorded, it wasn't done. But the corollary is also true: If it wasn't done, but was recorded, it's fraud. I make sure to delete parts of a template that were not done, not addressed, or not needed.

5. Technology is a tool that I utilize for patient care; it does not and should not replace the fundamentals of patient care, or common sense for that matter. A long and impressive looking office note with no substance helps no one. If an acute visit, for example, only needs a short note, I will only free text a short note.

6. I try to never complain about the EHR to the patient and try to explain and show how the use of the EHR can improve patient care. Getting the patient to look at something on the monitor such as the tracking of blood pressures, for example, is an excellent way to do just that.

A study in the Canadian Family Physician found that there was a correlation between patient satisfaction and their perception of the doctor's skill with the EHR software. Also, patients who felt the office was positive about EHR use were also more likely to be happy with the visit.

Change is never easy. As Woodrow Wilson said, "If you want to make enemies, try to change something."

It's in the best interests of our patients to try and get along with the EHR. If I've been able to do it, anyone should be able to as well.

I think the real challenge for the future is trying to figure out the best way to combine the tech-savvy expertise of many young physicians with the excellent communication skills of many tech-unsavvy older physicians. I know I can teach young physicians a lot about communication skills, and I know they can teach me a lot about technology.

I love the following quote by Michael Kirsch, MD: "Patients admire Dr. House's diagnostic acumen, but many still want Marcus Welby as their own doctor."

That's exactly what I want when I see my own doctors, as a patient.

Regarding #4 above:

"…it's an advantage and a disadvantage for patients/families and others to easily read records, compared to hand-written notes from "the old days." Medicolegally if it wasn't recorded it wasn't done. But the corollary is also true: If it wasn't done, but was recorded, it's fraud. Always make sure to delete parts of a template that were not done, not addressed, or not needed."

I have been a patient several times over the years and have accessed my own medical records.

I'm disillusioned when parts of the medical record document things that were not done.

Also, while there is considerable controversy regarding whether patients or families should ever be allowed to discretely record clinical encounters, it's always best, given readily available technology, to assume an encounter is being recorded.

It would be indefensible if such recordings were allowed during litigation and confirmed fraudulent documentation, perhaps at times, solely to increase reimbursement.

When to retire?

After many years of working, this becomes something for all to consider.

Physicians currently have no mandatory retirement age, regardless of specialty. The American Medical Association (AMA) estimates about 30% of the current physician workforce is greater than 65 years old. Whether or not there should be a mandatory retirement age for physicians is an ongoing hotly debated topic.

However, the AMA also predicts a significant shortage of physicians in the next decade or so.

Many feel this anticipated shortage will discourage healthcare organizations from using cognitive and functional evaluation tools to screen elderly physicians, to encourage and allow existing physicians to remain in practice for as long as possible.

I have known many physicians who have continued to see patients well into their 80s.

I will not be one such physician.

I knew an ophthalmologist, years ago, who was still an effective clinician at age 86 (due to his long-term memory), but whose family finally convinced him to retire when he got lost driving home from work, twice.

My grandfather continued to practice with metastatic prostate cancer until he became too symptomatic and weak to see patients. I can't remember if he ever officially retired. He died months later.

However, many of my medical school classmates and fellow residency graduates have already retired.

My dentist, whom I have seen for 29 years and is my age, recently announced his retirement.

My family doctor, whom I have seen for over 25 years and is my age, recently announced his retirement as well.

All these announcements always take me aback.

Aren't they too young to retire?

My wife has stated "you won't know what to do with yourself if you retire."

I don't have these same concerns.

John Chase MD, in his excellent book, "*You What?!*" makes some recommendations for physicians regarding this issue and it's applicable to most careers.

He advises you should continue to work if you still enjoy what you are doing, but goes on to recommend retiring when:

1. *you are still valued, but not yet pitied.*

and…

2. *when you have enough, and you have just about had enough.*

I continue to enjoy practicing on most days, but admittedly, after some days, have just about had enough.

I'm sure I'm still valued, but "when you have enough," given the world in which we live, is possibly the hardest question to feel confident in trying to answer.

A colleague recently reminded me of the social security life-expectancy calculator.

I entered my profile.

The result was a little depressing.

So…I'll continue to thoughtfully ponder when to retire from medicine.

On an even more personal level

"As for inflicting our sorrow on other people, one does not want to go around blathering and crying all the time. But perhaps it is our gift to others to trust them enough to share our feelings with them. It may help them deal with some of their own."-Martha Whitmore Hickman

My daughter, Ellie, and her mother had a truly wonderful relationship. Sadly, she and I witnessed her mom's cardiac arrest on June 18th, 2015.

While grieving, she wrote this:

Ecclesiastes 3:11-12-- "He has made everything beautiful in its time. He has also set eternity in the human hearts, yet no one can fathom what God has done from beginning to end. I know that there is nothing better for people than to be happy and to do good while they live."

Quite frankly, death sucks.

There is truly no other loss or devastation equal to that of the passing of a loved one. Whether you saw it creeping up slowly in the form of a slowly debilitating illness, or it appeared out of nowhere as a sudden, tragic event, it sucks.

Humans were not placed on this Earth to die. We were created to have dreams and make plans and forge relationships and pursue as many experiences as possible that the world has to offer. So, when something happens to throw all these things out of line, the entire world seems off kilter. Nothing can ever be back right how it was. In the depths of grief, it feels as if you are being struck again and again with massive waves, barely able to keep your head above water long enough to gasp for air before the next wave crashes over you.

When you can get your head above water again, it still isn't that great up there. Everything is out of focus and seemingly normal air can suddenly make your lungs burn. The most tedious and insignificant daily tasks are suddenly insurmountable challenges. People will say the most astonishing things to you in the guise of cheering you up. And the person you want to talk about these new life developments is no longer there.

And it sucks. So much.

When grieving the loss of one of the most important people in your life, it is utterly frustrating and downright unhelpful to have people tell you that they know exactly how you feel, or that they're shocked and sad for you, or that you should look at the bright side of your situation. People throw around phrases like "I'm so depressed," or "I feel like I'm dying" in everyday conversation without a second thought. People you meet will unknowingly release a river of emotion inside you with questions like how your summer was or how your family is doing. Any sort of human interaction is now a gamble, and you take your chances with those grief waves every morning when you wake up.

What no one ever tells you is that it's important to spend time in those depths of grief. This incredible loss is now a huge part of your life, and there's simply no avoiding that fact. Allowing yourself to feel those deep cuts in the very center of your being and having a good long cry about it can be very therapeutic in and of itself.

The key is to not get stuck in those depths. While life will never be the same again and may never seem nearly as amazing as it once was with your loved one, the sun will continue to rise day after day. As incredible as it may seem, the rest of the world will continue to function even though your entire personal world came crashing to pieces all around you. Like I said before, humans were put on this Earth to live. Not simply exist, not just go through the motions and trudge along day by day, but to go out and seize each day like the gift it truly is. You now understand better than anyone else that life is short, and life is precious.

So go and live it. Go to church, read inspirational quotes on the internet, go to the gym, do whatever it is you need to do to grant yourself even the smallest bit of internal relief. Forgive those who don't understand how they can hurt you with the smallest remarks. Learn to appreciate even the tiniest bit of sunshine in your day, even if it's something as small as having a great sandwich for lunch or securing the perfect parking spot. Realize that life is hard and unfair and sad, but at the same time it is so worth living to its fullest extent.

Allow yourself to visit that dark, horrible place and feel all those feelings, just don't make that place your home.

Prior to her death, a home in our neighborhood had been a total loss due to a fire. The homeowner was a friend and a firefighter.

Neighbors would comment how ironic it was for the home of a firefighter to have burned down.

For quite a while, I ruminated over thinking many must have thought it was ironic for her to have died suddenly in the home of a doctor.

It was my sister's birthday, and we had called earlier in the evening with our good wishes. Other than Tom, who went to a movie with a friend, we were all just home watching TV.

Tori was on the couch with our toy-poodle, Dwight, on her lap.

I was nine days post-op from a hip replacement, doing well, and on a recliner next to the couch.

Ellie was on the other side of the room, in a loveseat, and said, "Mom, are you alright?"

I looked over.

Dwight was still on her lap, but she had slumped over and wasn't moving.

She was unresponsive and without a pulse.

I started CPR--Ellie called 911--EMS arrived in 8 minutes.

I was finally allowed to see her in the emergency room when she had stabilized.

She had been in electromechanical dissociation for about 30 minutes.

She had decerebrate posturing.

After four days of observation and tests, life support was withdrawn to allow natural death.

We will all introspectively replay the events of those four days, intermittently, for the rest of our lives.

More on dealing with loss/grief

In the foreword to *A Grief Observed* by C.S. Lewis, Madeleine L'Engle notes, *"But when two people marry, each one has to accept that one of them will die before the other."*

However, this truth is usually never a significant part of a couple's psyche until old age or until one has been given a terminal diagnosis.

And, as C.S. Lewis notes, *"It's different when it happens to you, not to others, and is reality, not imaginary."*

This will be a brief review of my journey through loss, grief, and bereavement.

Only Ellie and Tom can chronicle theirs.

They lost a remarkable mother and their initial counsel for basically everything, because they knew she would always give them her undivided attention and she was wise beyond her years.

She was also a much beloved pediatric nurse practitioner in our community.

I did not always say or do the right things. I should have sought counseling for us, individually and as a family. I failed to either initiate or follow-through on many much-needed discussions.

They had to navigate much on their own because I was not always "there."

However, some great friends and extended family members were there for them.

I know I could have done better.

I'll always have some regrets regarding this period.

An association between bereavement and an increased mortality risk, due to multiple causes, is well known.

Suicide is one such cause.

Many contemplate suicide while grieving.

Although I never contemplated suicide, I did often think dying would have been a more comfortable route.

Years prior, we had agreed that we were fine with cremation.

"You don't have a soul. You have a body. You are a soul."- C.S. Lewis

We had previously completed advance directives and living wills.

I just never envisioned needing to invoke hers or do funeral home arrangements since I was nine years older.

We had wonderful neighbors and friends.

So many supported us in the initial weeks by checking in, bringing food, assisting with the memorial service, and setting up a memorial fund in her name.

My in-laws and brother-in-law lived locally.

They were great and we supported each other as best as we could but they were also navigating through their own grief after losing a daughter and a sister.

Most of our visits either included or ended with tears.

My mom and siblings phoned frequently, and their calls were always appreciated. I would usually just report we were all doing okay.

My sister and her wife helped with many things, including sorting through all her clothing and shoes. Most was donated to *Goodwill*.

I'm not sure when I would have been able to do the same.

"Bereavement is a darkness unknown to the imagination of the unbereaved."-Iris Murdoch

"Everyone can master a grief but he that has it."-William Shakespeare

I wasn't sleeping well. I would intermittently be sort of fine, then sad, then mad, and then overwhelmed. I felt guilty for being the surviving parent.

She always had a healthy lifestyle.

I resented others her age, or older, who didn't have a healthy lifestyle and were still alive. I begrudged other happy couples; why were they so fortunate to still have each other?

We had divided most household chores over our twenty-seven years together, but it became apparent that her chores-- shopping for groceries and household items, setting up and keeping track of appointments, deadlines, etc., for our family- -were the chores that really mattered.

Looking through her day planner, which I was never previously "allowed" to do, took my breath away.

While doing the dishes and taking out the trash were necessary, keeping the cars cleaned and stomping on mole tracks in our yard, some of my other "important" chores, were, appropriately, no longer a priority.

"No one ever told me that grief felt so like fear."-C.S. Lewis

I had many fears.

I was worried about finances, especially due to college expenses, so the three of us met with my financial advisor to review and plan.

I was worried about dying soon so I met with my neighbor, who was an attorney, to update my will.

I was worried about all her jewelry being stolen, so I procured a safety deposit box at the bank.

Our home was oppressively sad.

I felt the most "normal" away from our home.

I think the same was true for Ellie and Tom.

In the evenings we would watch episode after episode of *Seinfeld* re-runs.

It was much-needed comic relief and I'll always be grateful for this sitcom.

It was soon time for both to head back to college.

Ellie for her 2nd year at the University of Virginia and Tom for his junior year at Stetson University.

After they were gone, our home became even more suffocatingly sad.

Although Dwight had always been primarily attached to her, he sensed I was struggling and literally never left my side.

I finally considered counseling through the employee assistance program but got annoyed at the individual taking my intake information over the phone and decided to "f--k it, I can do this on my own."

This was another poor decision.

Thankfully…I eventually began to make better decisions.

I started to read more again.

Two especially helpful books were *A Grief Observed* by C.S. Lewis, given to me by a close friend from medical school, and *Healing After Loss* by Martha Whitmore Hickman, which appeared on my work desk with a wonderful, uplifting, un-signed note.

I reached out to a second cousin who had lost his wife years prior.

We hadn't spoken for a long time, but I appreciated his words of encouragement and being able to review my fears, concerns, and struggles.

I found a wonderful website, *"Lost Without Her,"* by Mark Oborn (lost-without-her.com).

His wife, Claire, had also died suddenly in her 40s and he therefore instantly became a widower-father as well.

"Whoever survives a test, whatever it may be, must tell the story. That is his duty."-Elie Wiesel

"Other people are going to find healing in your wounds. Your greatest life messages and your most effective ministry will come out of your deepest hurts."-Pastor Rich Warren

"God's desire is for us to use our painful life events to carry his message of hope, grace, forgiveness and mercy."-Author unknown

I started to put my thoughts down in a journal.

I then started a blog on day # 61 after her death-*Life without T* (wtslwt.blogspot.com).

Blog entry-August 22, 2015:

"It's day 61 since my wife died.

It continues to be a day of emotions that are all over the place.

I went to a men's group this morning sponsored by a local church that discussed the importance of men having relationships with other men to hold them accountable in life.

While there was some useful information, I found myself having to frequently talk myself out of crying whenever someone would mention the word "wife."

I recently came across a blog entitled "Lost without Her" …One entry ends with a reminder of how the authors wife would want him to spend the rest of his time on earth. She would want him to "smile, open his eyes, love and go on."

It's been my mantra today.

It helps to a degree but still doesn't stop the waves of emotion.

It does seem to keep me from drowning, however, and that's a good start."

I started to attend a weekly men's bible study group, thanks to an invite from a friend. I also participated in an 8-week support group at a local church for those *"Walking the Mourner's Path."*

I stopped wearing my wedding band after about five months.

Blog entry-November 9th, 2015:

"Accept what is, let go of what was, and have faith in what will be."-Sonia Ricotti

I was blessed with a wonderful wife and two awesome children.

Our wedding vows included the classic phrase "until death do us part."

The symbol of our marriage, my wedding band, was always something that I was so proud to wear.

The wedding band also held up through too numerous to count hours of yard work, dishes, and sports over the years.

T's death parted us 140 days ago, but I couldn't let go of the band on my finger until a few days ago.

It's now in my bedside table."

Everything began to slowly improve.

"The strength, courage and qualities I have found within myself through the process of grief is unparalleled to what I ever knew existed."-Melissa Wilder Joyce

My fears started to abate.

I reconnected more positively with my family and friends.

The times Ellie, Tom and I spent together were of much better quality.

"Shrines have their place but are poor backgrounds for life in the present moment."-Martha Whitmore Hickman

I sold our home, rented a storage unit for the bulk of our possessions, and moved into a two-bedroom apartment.

I agonized for a long time over what do with her ashes as we had never discussed such details.

We were never a fan of memorial parks or memorial walls.

We also thought keeping a loved-one's ashes in the home or on a mantel, as was spoofed in one of our favorite movies, *Meet the Parents,* was silly.

I finally awakened to what I thought we should do, and Ellie, Tom and her parents agreed.

We had experienced many awesome, laughter-filled family vacations over the years at the beach.

Ellie, Tom, and I scattered her ashes there, about four years after she had died.

I copied scripture or quotes onto sticky notes. I kept them in my wallet, or on my desk at work, to read when emotionally ambushed.

Here are some that consistently helped to console me:

"Rejoice always, pray continually, give thanks in all circumstances; this is God's will for you in Christ Jesus."-1 Thessalonians 5:16-18

"It is what it is."-Author unknown

"Remember that guy who gave up? No worries, neither does anyone else…"-Author unknown *"*

"Grief for things past that cannot be remedied will never benefit me. I will therefore commit myself to God and enjoy the present."-Joseph Hall

"This is the only day I have for sure; may I use it well."-Martha Whitmore Hickman

"No matter how you feel--get up, dress up, show up and never give up."-Regina Brett

"When in doubt just take the next small step."-Paulo Coelho

"Every morning starts a new page in your story. Make it a great one today."-Doe Zantamata

"Don't let the sadness of your past, and the fear of your future, ruin the happiness of your present."-Author unknown

"Open your hand and heart to life as it is now."-Author unknown

"Life is too short for long pity parties. Get busy living or get busy dying."-from The Shawshank Redemption

"Those who died yesterday had plans for this morning. And those who died this morning had plans for tonight. Don't take life for granted. In the blink of an eye, everything can change. So, forgive often and love with a full heart. You never know when you may not have that chance again."-Amanda Rose

"You can honor your past, you can treasure your past, you can and should love your past, but you don't have to live in the past."-Author unknown

"I like to remind myself that my track record for getting through bad days so far is 100%, and that's pretty good."-Author unknown

"Your feelings of loss don't disappear, but they soften as you know the person who died will never be forgotten but that you can and will move forward in your life."-Alan Wolfelt

"The ache is always there, but one day not the emptiness because to nurture the emptiness, to take solace in it, is to disrespect the gift of life."-Dean Koontz

*"Life is short, live it. Love is rare, grab it. Anger is bad, dump it. Fear is awful, face it. Memories are sweet, cherish it."-*Author unknown

*"If you are alive in the morning you can continue to work on it; if not, you didn't need to finish it anyway."-*Author unknown

*"Our greatest accomplishment is not in never failing, but in rising every time we fall."-*Confucius

*"The best memorial to our loved one is to live our lives fully, one day at a time."-*Author unknown

*"Do not regret growing old--it's a privilege denied to many."-*Mark Twain

And finally, a quote I kept on my refrigerator and read every morning, for a few years:

*"Choose to live in Joy: Life goes by in the blink of an eye. It's too short to live upset, angry, resentful, or ungrateful. If you look for the good, you'll find it. Choose to be happy, to be at peace. Decide each day is going to be a great day and grab each moment and make the best of it. Refuse to let negative thoughts take root in your mind and refuse to let negative people and situations drag you down. Trust your journey and know that if you make a mistake, it's okay. See it as a lesson learned and keep moving forward. Spend less time worrying and more time being grateful for those who love you and all of life's goodness. Choose to live in joy!"-*Charity M. Richey-Bentley

---

Abraham Lincoln's mother died suddenly in 1818. He was nine years old. Years later, during the Civil War, he wrote the following letter to Fanny McCullough, the young daughter of a colleague, William McCullough, who had been killed in battle in December 1862:

"In this sad world of ours, sorrow comes to all; and, to the young, it comes with bitterest agony, because it takes them unawares. The older have learned to ever expect it. I am anxious to afford some alleviation of your present distress. Perfect relief is not possible, except with time. You cannot now realize that you will ever feel better. Is not this so? And yet it is a mistake. You are sure to be happy again. To know this, which is certainly true, will make you some less miserable now. I have had experiences enough to know what I say, and you need only to believe it, to feel better at once. The memory of your dear Father, instead of an agony, will yet be a sad sweet feeling in your heart, of a purer and holier sort than you have known before."

Lives are never the same after a loss, but his words are accurate.

Birthday and anniversary dates remain emotionally challenging to a degree and significant family milestones cause you to reflect more intensely, but you are sure to be happy again.

It takes time, but you become progressively more thankful for the life you shared than for the sadness of your loss.

An update, seven and one-half years later:

-Almost two years after Tori's death, I reluctantly decided to attend a Florida Academy of Family Physicians medical conference.

It was a beautiful Saturday, and I really didn't want to spend it indoors at a conference.

But I went and it was a great decision.

I can't recall one topic that was presented at the conference, but I ran into Jenni during a break.

We knew each other but had not crossed paths for many years.

We re-connected immediately.

Amid briefly catching up it was also apparent that we had both been through some life changing events.

We met for coffee the next Saturday.

We began to date.

We married a couple of years later.

We have blended two families, with five children, their spouses, significant others, and multiple pets, and I could not be more thankful.

-After college, Ellie and Tom went on to complete higher degrees of study. Ellie's now a Doctor of Veterinary Medicine and Tom's a Doctor of Physical Therapy.

Both are also in healthy, loving, long term relationships.

I could not be prouder or happier for them.

A few other quotes that have spoken to me over the years

"That's the thing about life; it's fragile, precious, and unpredictable and each day is a gift, not a given right."-Holly Butcher (In her essay, *"A bit of life advice from Hol,"* before she died from Ewing's sarcoma at age twenty-seven.)

"Try just enjoying and being in moments rather than capturing them through the screen of your phone. Life isn't meant to be lived through a screen nor is it about getting the perfect photo. Enjoy the bloody moment people! Stop trying to capture it for everyone else."-Holly Butcher

"Humility is the only lens through which great things can be seen--and once we have seen them, humility is the only posture possible." -Parker Palmer

"In general, we aren't learning much when our lips are moving."-Author unknown

"Delight in the gift of life and be grateful."-Parker Palmer

"The civility we need will not come from watching our tongues. It will come from honoring our differences."-Parker Palmer

"True humility is not thinking less of yourself. It's thinking of yourself, less."-Pastor Rich Warren

"Wholeness does not mean perfection; it means embracing brokenness as an integral part of life."-Parker Palmer

"You don't know how much time you've got on this Earth, so don't waste it being miserable."-Author unknown

"The laws of nature that dictate the sunset dictate our demise. But how we travel the arc between our own sunrise and sundown is ours to choose."-Author unknown

"We all have the same 86,400 seconds in a day. How we use them is ours to choose."-Author unknown

"Friendship is born when one person says to another, what, you too? I thought I was the only one."-C.S. Lewis

"Collect memories, not things."-Author unknown

"Prize being over having, experiences over material possessions."-Author unknown

"The most beautiful things in life are not things. They're people and places and memories and pictures. They're feelings and moments and smiles and laughter."-Author unknown

"The real enemy is arrogance…whether it's arrogance about race, wealth, gender, sex, or religion, it is all decidedly un-American. Personally, I am going to work on my arrogance and try to become a better citizen of this country. Those who have served, fought, and died for my right to become a better American deserve no less of me."-Chester Buckenmaier III, MD, COL (ret), MC, USA

Final Thoughts

"The only way to become whole is to put our arms lovingly around-everything-we know ourselves to be: self-serving and generous, spiteful and compassionate cowardly and courageous, treacherous and trustworthy."-Parker Palmer

While I prefer for others to think I've only exemplified the admirable qualities, I acknowledge that I've been all the above, at times, over the course of my life.

Internationally acclaimed author, Bronnie Ware, spent years working in palliative care. She first noted, in a 2009 blog entry, five common themes that anguished those who expressed their feelings prior to death:

"1. I wish I'd had the courage to live a life true to myself, not the life others expected of me. 2. I wish I didn't work so hard. 3. I wish I'd had the courage to express my feelings. 4. I wish I had stayed in touch with my friends. 5. I wish that I had let myself be happier."

Number two is a much-needed reminder for many of us. It's important to maintain as good a balance as possible between your career and your family to avoid regrets, regarding this, later in life.

A few pet peeves:

1. Disability parking:

If you are not disabled, never use a disability parking placard unless you are the driver, and the disabled individual is with you in the car.

If you've been issued a disability placard or license plate, but are doing relatively well, possibly consider using a regular parking space.

For example, if you are currently able to walk briskly and unaided, carrying a satchel into your fitness center, do you really need to be taking up one of the few disability spaces that could be used by someone who has a more significant or symptomatic impairment?

2. Social media:

Posting intimate messages to a loved one, especially when living in the same house or even sharing the same bed.

Social media is engineered to be "seductive, irresistible and addictive." This possibly explains why many post things that should ideally only be shared in private.

After reading such a post, I always envision the following:

"Good morning honey, please look at Facebook now, before I say anything else or give you a card, because I've shared some intimate thoughts, meant just for you, so our friends can read, and, hopefully, like and comment."

3. Diminished respectful interactions:

Even the simple act of acknowledging someone when you cross paths. I always enjoy saying "HELLO" to anyone who keeps their head down, often scrolling through their phone.

Some occasionally say hello back, instead of looking startled, or annoyed, that I bothered them.

For anyone interested

I've enjoyed writing on varied topics over the years.

PUBLICATIONS:

- Sheahan WT, Sheahan TE. Elective Hip Arthroplasty: Which Surgical Approach is Optimal? Federal Practitioner. 2022; 39(4):186-189.
- Sheahan WT, Parvataneni HK. Asymptomatic but Time for a Hip Revision. Federal Practitioner. 2016 February;33(2): 47-51.
- Sheahan WT, Martinez SQ, Golden AG. Testosterone Replacement Therapy: Playing Catch-up with Patients. Federal Practitioner. 2015 June;32(6):26-31.
- Sheahan WT. My Word Column, Orlando Sentinel, June 18, 2014: Navigating our complicated health care.
- Sheahan WT. My Word Column, Orlando Sentinel, March 1, 2014: Ins and Outs of applying for college.
- Sheahan WT. Advanced Parkinson Disease-It's More Than Just a Tremor. Federal Practitioner. 2013 December; 30 (12):14-18.
- Sheahan WT. Orlando Sentinel, December 25, 2013: Life before dementia.
- Sheahan WT. Letters to the Editor: Benzodiazepine Use and Hip Fractures in Older Adults. Am Fam Physician. 2013 Dec 1; 88 (11): 728.
- Sheahan WT. Orlando Sentinel, September 26, 2013: Coaches and life's lessons.
- Sheahan WT. Bringing the EHR into the Physician-Patient Relationship, Physicians Practice (www.physicianspractice.com) July 23, 2012.
- Sheahan WT. Orlando Sentinel, June 20, 2012: A Soccer controversy.

- Sheahan WT. Orlando Sentinel, November 28, 2011: Competitive, clean programs should be the focus of athletics.
- Sheahan WT. Can inappropriate MRI be stopped? The American Family Physician Community Blog, May 22, 2011.
- Sheahan WT. Patients Say the Darndest Things #3. ISBN 978-1-60910-016-2; 2009
- Sheahan WT. Patients Say the Darndest Things # 2. ISBN 1-59113-907-4; 2006
- Sheahan WT. Orlando Sentinel, June 4, 2005: Nick Anderson's legacy.
- Sheahan WT. Patients Say the Darndest Things. ISBN 1-59113-397-1; 2003
- Sheahan WT. It's just all in his head. Patient Care, Case and Comment, September 2003; 37:80-84.
- Sheahan WT. When the snowbirds return. Medical Economics 2003; 80(9):105.
- Sheahan WT. My Word Column, Orlando Sentinel, February 6, 2003: Physician: Balance alternative, traditional medicine.
- Sheahan WT. What an FP's week is really like. Medical Economics 2003; 80(1):36-38.
- Sheahan WT. Running late. Medical Economics 2002; June 7; 79(11):94-97.
- Sheahan WT. CMEzzzzzzzzz. Medical Economics 2002: April 26; 79(8) 2002:50-53.
- Sheahan WT. I can't do my job. Patient Care, Case and Comment, February 28, 2002: 48-49.
- Sheahan WT. A limping 5-year-old boy. Patient Care, Case and Comment, November 15, 2001: 65-66.
- Sheahan WT. Take this patient's history- please. Medical Economics Web Exclusive (www.memag.com), June 18, 2001.

- Sheahan WT. R&R in a hospital? Surely you jest. Medical Economics Web Exclusive (www.memag.com), February 5, 2001.
- Sheahan WT. Depression, deficits, and gynecomastia. Patient Care, Case and Comment, September 15, 2000: 146.
- Sheahan WT. My Word Column, Orlando Sentinel, September 6, 2000: What pills should go into bean soup?
- Sheahan WT. How to harmonize with PAs and NPs. Medical Economics 2000; 77(16):69-70.
- Sheahan WT. Syncope in a patient with aortic stenosis. Patient Care, Case and Comment, August 15, 2000: 115-116.
- Sheahan WT. My patient's car is his castle. Medical Economics 2000; 77(4):87-90.
- Sheahan WT. You can't be the right doctor for your family. Medical Economics 1999; 76(23):97-98.
- Sheahan WT. Anxiety and a severe headache. Patient Care, Case and Comment, September 30, 1999: 112.
- Sheahan WT. A locking sensation in the hip. Patient Care, Case and Comment, September 15, 1999: 281-284.
- Wright, AM, Rexrode CR, Hoffman RH, Lustig MR, Sheahan WT, King JG, Marsland DW. Selected Disorders of the Respiratory System. Family Medicine: Principles and Practice, 4th ed., Taylor RB (editor), New York, NY. Springer-Verlag, 1995.

9 798885 312011